Lower Your
Blood Sugar
⌘ Bible ⌘

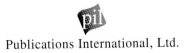

Publications International, Ltd.

Pictured on the front cover: Tuna Steaks with Pineapple and Tomato Salsa *(page 134)*.

Pictured on the back cover *(clockwise from top):* Strawberry-Banana Granité *(page 188)*, Mediterranean Pita Pizzas *(page 242)* and Ham & Egg Breakfast Panini *(page 40)*.

Contributing Writers: Timothy Gower and Allison S. Zalay RD, LDN

Photography on pages 4, 8, 10, 11, 13, 14, 17 and 21 by Shutterstock.
Photography on page 21 by Dreamstime.

ISBN-13: 978-1-4508-6087-1
ISBN-10: 1-4508-6087-7

Library of Congress Control Number: 2012944211

Manufactured in China.

8 7 6 5 4 3 2 1

Publications International, Ltd.

CONTENTS

INTRODUCTION

What's the Big Deal About Blood Sugar?

It *is* a big deal—knowing how to control your blood sugar can help you manage your hunger, appetite, weight and health condition and lead a healthier life.

Pay Attention

It has become medical boilerplate: After just about every office visit, doctors give patients strict orders to eat right and exercise. We hear these cautions so often that it's easy to zone out and think, *Right, doc, whatever you say.... I wonder if I have time to stop for a cheeseburger on the way back to work....* The truth is, though, that we are becoming an overweight and obese population and it is time to start paying attention to our health.

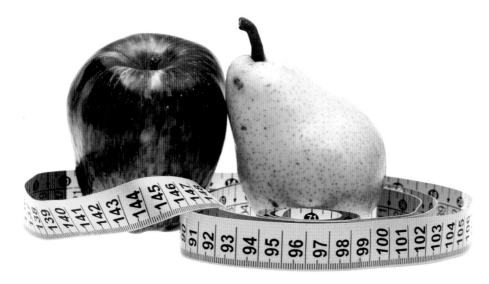

Some Statistics

Just how tubby have we become? About 65 percent of Americans are overweight, with 30 percent considered obese. For perspective, the Centers for Disease Control and Prevention define a person who is 5 feet 4 inches tall and weighs more than 145 pounds as overweight; someone who is the same height and weighs more than 174 pounds is considered obese. Compare those statistics to the late 1970s, when fewer than half of Americans were overweight and just 15 percent were obese. What's more, the number of Americans who are more than 100 pounds overweight quadrupled between 1986 and 2000.

Obesity isn't the only epidemic going on in this country. About 20.8 million Americans—roughly 7 percent of the population—have diabetes. Furthermore, an additional 6.2 million Americans have diabetes but don't know it. And this problem isn't going away anytime soon. About 1.5 million new cases of diabetes are diagnosed each year in Americans aged 20 years and older.

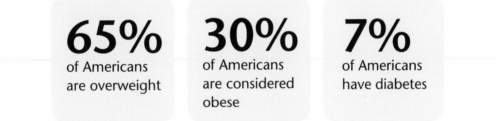

65%
of Americans
are overweight

30%
of Americans
are considered
obese

7%
of Americans
have diabetes

What is Diabetes?

There are two types of diabetes mellitus: type 1 insulin-dependent diabetes, also known as juvenile diabetes, and type 2 diabetes, formerly known as non-insulin dependent diabetes mellitus or adult-onset diabetes.

About 90 percent of all people with diabetes in the United States have type 2 diabetes. That adds up to more than 16 million Americans, or enough people to populate New York City—twice.

The Obesity-Diabetes Connection

Since type 2 diabetes is more common, the question then is, does obesity cause diabetes? Most doctors believe that, yes, obesity is an important cause of diabetes. For example, Mississippi is the state with the highest rate of obesity at 25.9 percent of the state's population (and 28 percent of adults). It also has the highest rate of diabetes (11 percent). Coincidence?

The next question then becomes, how much does being overweight increase the risk of type 2 diabetes? Imagine two men, both 5 feet 10 inches tall. The first weighs 167 pounds, while the other tips the scales at 209 pounds. The second man is five times more likely to develop type 2 diabetes, according to a 2005 Harvard University study.

Knowledge is Power

It's time to start paying more attention to food and nutrition,

Are You Overweight?

Stepping on the scale doesn't tell the whole story. Doctors use body mass index (BMI) to determine whether a person's weight is proportionate to their height. If your BMI falls between 25 and 29, you're overweight. If it's 30 or higher, you are considered obese.

Here's how to calculate your BMI:

1) Weigh yourself first thing in the morning without clothes.

2) Confirm your height in inches.

3) Multiply your weight in pounds by 700.

4) Divide the result in step 3 by your height in inches.

5) Divide the result in step 4 by your height in inches again.

The resulting number is your BMI.

taking control and begin putting health first! Whether you are watching your weight, newly diagnosed or have been living with diabetes for years, you can use this book as a guide to eating your favorite foods with a healthy twist.

Just the Basics

Let's start with a basic understanding of how the body functions and how it is affected by food.

After a meal, the body breaks down food into glucose during digestion. The term "blood glucose" is often used interchangeably with "blood sugar," as glucose is a simple form of sugar. Glucose provides the energy for every function the body performs from walking and lifting weights to sleeping.

Excess glucose that isn't used for energy right away is stored in the muscle, liver and fat tissues for later use. Insulin is a hormone that is responsible for taking the glucose that has been released into the bloodstream after digestion and storing it in the muscle, liver and fat cells as glycogen.

What is Insulin?

If glucose could simply slip into the body's cells on its own, there would be no such thing as diabetes, and you could be out working in the garden or playing with the kids instead of reading this book. However, glucose needs assistance from insulin, which acts like a doorman, unlocking cells so that glucose can enter and be used as fuel.

The pancreas, a five-inch organ tucked under the stomach, produces a pair of hormones, insulin and glucagon, that regulate glucose levels in the blood to help maintain stable blood sugar levels at all times. Hormones are the body's expediters, zipping around from one organ to another as needed. When glucose levels begin to rise in the blood, the pancreas cranks out insulin to help get glucose into cells. When blood sugar levels drop too low, the pancreas produces glucagon, which travels to the liver with orders to convert some glycogen back into glucose, then release it into the blood.

For those with type 1 diabetes, the pancreas is not able to produce insulin. Consequently, blood glucose produced by digestion continues to circulate in the bloodstream. In type 2 diabetes, the pancreas produces insulin but the muscle, liver and fat cells that should accept the glucose from insulin do not function properly and won't accept it, leaving excess glucose in the bloodstream. This is known as insulin resistance. Strong associations have been found between insulin resistance and being overweight or obese.

Breaking It Down

Calories are the fuel that the body uses as energy. They come from four main sources—carbohydrates, protein, fat and alcohol—and each affect blood glucose levels differently. Most foods provide calories from more than one source, so it's important to look at the nutrition information on food packages for a full breakdown.

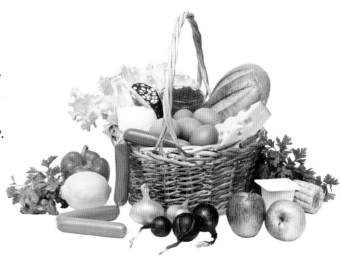

Carbohydrates

Humans can burn both fat and protein as fuel and muscle mass prefers fatty acids. But the preferred source of energy of both body and brain are carbohydrates, which break down into glucose.

You know that carbohydrates are sugars and starches found in fruits, vegetables and grains. While that's true, it's hardly the whole picture, since junk food like soda pop, pizza, potato chips and cupcakes are also packed with carbs. Clearly, some carbohydrate-rich foods are healthier than others. But once food has been digested, your body can't tell whether a carbohydrate came from a banana or a candy bar. Carbohydrates all become glucose, regardless of their source.

Carbohydrates make up approximately half of the calories we consume, and are also the greatest contributor to our blood glucose levels. Digestion breaks down carbohydrates easily and rapidly, which is why eating white bread causes a rapid spike in blood sugar levels.

During digestion, the body converts carbohydrates into glucose. After a meal that contains carbohydrates, the glucose is quickly absorbed by body cells. Some is immediately used for energy, while the rest is placed into short-term storage—in the form of glycogen—primarily in the liver and muscle mass. When you eat more carbohydrates than you need for immediate energy and short-term reserve in the liver and muscles, your body converts glucose into fat, which is sent to long-term storage, usually in the belly, butt and thighs.

What Exactly are Carbohydrates?

Potatoes and pinto beans. Carrots and cauliflower. Rye bread and rock candy. Juice and soda pop. These foods have one thing in common: They're all sources of carbohydrates. They come in all shapes and sizes. They're found in fruits, vegetables, grains, beans, dairy products and just about everything other than meat, fish or fat. Broadly speaking, carbohydrates fall into three categories:

Sugars

The word "sugar" may make you think of the white granules you spoon into coffee or add to baked goods, but the sweet stuff comes in many varieties. Sugars are the simplest form of carbohydrates and include sucrose (found in table sugar and some fruits and vegetables), fructose (found in fruit and honey) and lactose (found in milk), among others.

Eliminating sugar from your diet isn't fun—and it's impractical, too. In fact, registered dietitians say there is no need—make that no way—to follow a "diabetes diet," since there is no such thing. Instead, you can help control your glucose levels by following a balanced meal plan consisting of nutritious foods and occasional indulgences, made up of enough calories to keep your engine running and maintain a healthy weight (or few enough to shed pounds if you're lugging around too many).

That's not to say that the amount of sugar you consume doesn't matter. If you live on candy and soda, chances are you will have pretty lousy glucose control. But remember, sugars are carbohydrates, and a carb is a carb is a carb once it hits your gut—so to your body they are all sources of glucose. Studies in the 1990s determined that the key to controlling blood sugar is to avoid consuming too many carbohydrates, period.

So while most of the carbohydrates in your diet should come from healthy sources, such as fruits, vegetables and whole grains, you can make room for a sweet treat now and then. Your doctor, registered dietitian or diabetes educator will help you determine what daily total amount of carbohydrates is healthy for you. Bottom line: You can have your cake and eat it too, as long as you curb your carbs in your meals and throughout the day.

Starches

Although they consist of sugar units, the complex structure of starches makes them a distinct type of carbohydrate. (In fact, nutrition professionals used to call starches "complex carbohydrates," though the term has fallen out of favor.) The large size of starch molecules also sets them apart from sugars; they're too big for taste bud receptors on the tongue, which is why starches usually don't taste sweet. Starchy foods include potatoes, bread, pasta and rice.

It is important to go with the (whole) grain. Many people grew up eating white bread and white pasta, but wheat isn't white. White flour is produced by grinding wheat to remove the sturdy outer layers of the grain, known as the bran and germ. Unfortunately, this refining process not only strips away the bran and germ, but also removes lots of fiber, vitamins (especially vitamins B and E) and minerals, too. The same thing happens when rice is processed to make it pearly white.

The U.S. government requires commercial bakers to enrich their products, restoring some of the nutrients lost in refining. But some nutrition professionals believe that the body is better able to absorb and use naturally occurring vitamins and minerals. What's more, enrichment does not return the countless micronutrients found in grains to the finished product.

Whole grain breads, pasta and rice are made with the entire grain, and have a bolder taste and chewier texture than most of their paler cousins. Over time, you may find that white bread and other refined grains taste bland. Beware of imitators: Some commercial bakeries sell "wheat" bread that is simply white bread that has been dyed brown. Pasta makers sometimes dye pasta brown, too, to make it appear healthier. Look for the words "whole grain" or "whole wheat" on packages.

Fiber

Your grandma called it "roughage." Your gut calls it "indigestible." Fiber is made up of an intricate array of sugar molecules like starch, but these sugar molecules aren't absorbed into the bloodstream because the body lacks enzymes to break them down. Even though fiber isn't technically a nutrient, it does plenty of good.

Dietary fiber is a key component to the success in any diet. Fiber has been proven effective in disease prevention, weight loss and blood glucose control. It's naturally present in plants and therefore is a major nutritional component of fruits, vegetables, beans, nuts, seeds and whole grains. While many processed food products do have some added fiber, the best sources are natural, unrefined foods—common ingredients in many of the recipes in this book.

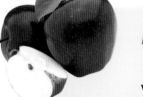

Five Ways to Increase the Fiber in Your Diet

1. *Start out strong.* Choose a high-fiber hot cereal with fruit for breakfast.

2. *Switch to whole grains.* Try brown rice, whole grain pastas and breads.

3. *Eat the whole fruit.* The fiber is in the peel and the pulp. Foods with edible seeds, such as berries, are fiber filled, too.

4. *Don't peel.* Paring off the skin of potatoes or other vegetables and fruits strips away fiber and nutrients, so leave it on. Corn and beans have edible skin, too.

5. *Get big on beans.* Full of fiber, protein, B vitamins and other nutrients, beans and lentils belong on any healthy menu. Eat beans or lentils three times a week.

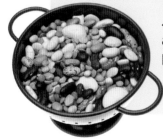

INTRODUCTION

Dietary fiber slows down the process of digestion, which gives the brain time to receive the message that the stomach is full. Also, fiber slows down the breakdown of food to glucose, moderating the blood glucose rise that occurs after any meal.

There are two types of dietary fiber, insoluble and soluble fiber, and both play an important role in weight loss. Insoluble fiber increases the bulk in the stomach, while soluble fiber slows down the digestive processes. As a result, you feel fuller from a smaller amount of food for an extended period of time.

Most of the fiber we consume is insoluble fiber. This type of fiber increases the weight and size of your stool, which allows regular bowel movements to occur, preventing constipation and aiding in digestive health. If you want to increase the fiber to your diet, just be cautious not to add too much too quickly, or to increase the amount of fiber in your diet without increasing your water intake. A drastic increase of fiber in the diet can cause abdominal discomfort, gas and constipation.

Soluble fiber—commonly found in beans, oats, and the peels of apples—absorbs water, providing a feeling of fullness as you eat, which helps you avoid overeating. It also slows down the digestive processes, helping to delay the blood glucose response after a meal.

Soluble fiber plays an important role in heart health, too. When bound to water, soluble fiber forms a gel-like substance in the digestive tract that absorbs cholesterol and carries it out of the body. This reduces blood cholesterol levels, helping to reduce the risk of heart disease.

Fiber supplements are an effective way to add bulk to your diet, but it is better to get fiber from foods. High-fiber pills, powders and snacks contain natural substances such as psyllium seed husks, which come from a type of plantain, but fiber-rich foods are also excellent sources of vitamins and minerals. Also, fiber supplements are commonly used as laxatives, so it's important to use them only as directed.

High-Fiber Fruits and Vegetables
(per 1 cup, unless otherwise indicated)

Avocado, cubed	10g
Green peas	9g
Raspberries	8g
Acorn squash	6g
Pear, large with skin	6g
Apple, large with skin	5g
Corn	5g
Potato, medium, baked with skin	5g
Asparagus	4g
Carrot	4g
Orange	4g
Spinach, cooked	4g
Strawberries	4g
Banana, medium	3g
Broccoli	2g
Grapefruit, ½ of whole fruit	2g

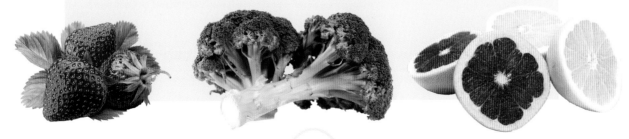

INTRODUCTION

Protein

Protein is essential for many cell functions, including providing structure and shape to cells. During digestion, protein breaks down into amino acids, which construct and repair muscles, organs and other body tissues. It also can be converted to glucose for use as energy when carbohydrates are low in supply.

Protein—found in products such as lean meats, fish, soy, dairy products, beans and nuts—is digested comparatively slowly, so eating foods with a significant amount of protein makes you feel full sooner and satisfied longer after eating. Additionally, when protein is eaten with carbohydrates, the protein delays the blood glucose response.

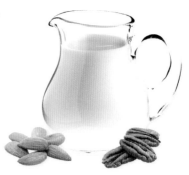

Although protein is very important, you probably don't need to add more to your diet. The fact is, most Americans consume far more protein than the body needs for the ongoing job of rebuilding muscle and other tissue.

Fat

There is a lot of speculation on where fat fits within the diet. For many years, fat was considered to be bad and something to be restricted, but this is not necessarily true. While fat does contribute more calories than equivalent amounts of carbohydrates or protein, certain types of fat have been proven to have health benefits.

The types of fats to limit are saturated fats and trans fats, commonly found in butter, cheeses, meats and other animal products. These types of fats have been found to increase levels of LDL cholesterol (the "bad" cholesterol) in the body and therefore are strongly connected to the risk of heart disease. On the other hand, monounsaturated fats and polyunsaturated fats—present in avocados, vegetable oils and fish—have been found to improve heart health by decreasing LDL cholesterol levels in the body, as well as reducing inflammation.

There is no need to eliminate fat from your diet, but do watch the type and amount consumed as it's a large source of calories. Replace foods in your diet that may be high in saturated or trans fats with those that are higher in unsaturated fats. For example, sauté your vegetables in olive oil instead of butter, and replace some meat with fish that is higher in unsaturated fats, such as salmon.

Substituting Good Fats for Bad Fats

1. Cook with olive oil. If you need flavorless oil, try canola or grapeseed oil. If the recipe requires the rich taste of butter, you can usually replace half of it with oil without compromising the flavor.

2. Prepare it yourself. Store-bought prepared salad dressings, marinades and sauces can be loaded with unhealthy fats, sugar, sodium and preservatives. Make a simple vinaigrette or marinade with olive oil, or just pass a good quality vinegar and olive oil at the table.

3. Avoid processed meat. It is not only loaded with sodium, it may also be high in fat.

4. Choose low-fat dairy. Drink low-fat milk and cook with low-fat dairy products. Watch out for cheese, as it can contribute a lot of saturated fat to your diet. Try using small amounts of full-flavored cheeses like Parmesan or feta.

5. Cook at home. It is no secret that foods prepared at restaurants are not good for us; they're loaded with hidden undesirable ingredients and the portion sizes are huge! Eating out often results in a higher intake of fat, carbohydrates, sodium and calories.

Not All Fat is the Same

There are four basic types of fat:

- **Saturated fat.** Fat molecules are made up of chains of carbon atoms with attached pairs of hydrogen atoms. Scientists say this form of fat is saturated because each molecule is packed with hydrogen atoms. For complex chemical, biological and anthropological reasons, many human beings (especially in the western hemisphere) find the taste of saturated fat to be exceptionally yummy. Whole milk, heavy cream, ice cream, butter, bacon and juicy steaks are all rich sources of saturated fat. Unfortunately, saturated fat also causes a rise in LDL cholesterol, the bad kind that lodges in arteries and increases the risk of cardiovascular disease—a disease strongly associated with diabetes.

- **Monounsaturated fat.** These fat molecules are missing one chain of hydrogen atoms ("mono" means "one"). Foods that are very high in monounsaturated fat are liquid at room temperature and include olive, nut and canola oils. Avocados and most varieties of nuts are good sources, too. Unlike the saturated variety, monounsaturated fats are good for you and your heart health, since they help lower LDL cholesterol levels.

- **Polyunsaturated fat.** Margarine, many kinds of vegetable oils (including corn oil) and fish are all sources of polyunsaturated fats, which are made up of molecules missing more than one pair of hydrogen atoms. While polyunsaturated fats do not receive bad press like saturated fat does, one type of polyunsaturated fat, omega-6 fatty acids, has been linked to health problems, including high blood pressure, an elevated risk for blood clotting and low levels of HDL ("good") cholesterol. On the other hand, the omega-3 fatty acids in fish oil appear to be beneficial for the heart. Evidence suggests that they reduce the risk of sudden cardiac death (which is caused by erratic heart rhythm), in addition to lowering cholesterol and triglycerides.

- **Trans fat.** This form of unsaturated fat has been chemically altered to prolong its shelf life, and shelves in your local supermarket are just where you'll find these fats. They are used heavily in commercial baking—many cookies, cakes, chips, crackers and pastries contain trans fats, and that's just the start. They are often used in frying and turn up in vegetable shortening and some margarines (especially the stick variety). You may appreciate a long shelf life when you discover an unopened bag of chips you left in the cupboard six months ago, but the convenience trans fats offer comes with a cost. Trans fat is chemically similar to saturated fat, so not surprisingly, it also raises LDL cholesterol.

What About Salt?

Hypertension, or high blood pressure, is a disease that is prevalent in diabetics and nondiabetics alike. High glucose levels can cause damage to the kidneys, which interferes with their ability to filter blood. This allows waste to pass back into circulation, which in turn increases your blood's volume and raises blood pressure.

What does this have to do with salt? Most of the sodium you eat comes from sodium chloride (table salt), which can cause blood pressure to rise in some people. There's no way of knowing whether your blood pressure will go through the roof if you consume too much sodium, so it's smart to consume less.

The human body only requires 400 milligrams of sodium, yet the typical American consumes more than 3,000 milligrams each day. The government recommends limiting sodium intake to 2,400 milligrams per day. This sounds like a lot, but it's equivalent to the sodium in about 1 teaspoon of table salt.

The salt shaker is only a small part of the problem. Processed foods get much of their flavor from sodium; Americans get an estimated 77 percent of their sodium from prepared or processed foods.

Shake the Salt Habit

Nutrition Professionals say that the human taste for salt can be unlearned. Cut back on high-sodium foods for a few weeks, and eventually your palate can adapt. Here are some strategies:

- *Look for the words "reduced sodium" or "no salt" on packages. You can always taste the food and add a small sprinkle of table salt if needed.*

- *If you buy canned foods that are swimming in a salty liquid or brine, rinse them to remove some sodium.*

- *Eat fresh produce when possible and cut back on processed or fast foods.*

- *Get creative with herbs and spices to add some zing to food that might otherwise taste bland without salt.*

- *Don't automatically add salt to a dish; taste it first—you may be pleasantly surprised. Do the same before adding salty condiments.*

- *At restaurants, ask if your meals can be prepared without monosodium glutamate (MSG) or high-sodium ingredients.*

Where does all the salt come from? Sodium is a stealth mineral. Salty-tasting foods to watch out for include fast-food meals, canned soups and vegetables (unless marked low- or no-sodium), frozen foods, breads, cookies, chips, crackers, breakfast cereals, condiments, pickles, seasonings and antacids.

Putting It All Together

When you eat something high in carbohydrates, your blood glucose will rise quickly. While all foods cause glucose levels to rise, carbohydrates have the swiftest impact, producing an increase in blood sugar within two hours of a meal. When carbohydrates are eaten along with some protein or fat, the blood glucose response is delayed. That is because fat and protein—which also break down into glucose—go through many more steps at the cellular level before this occurs and thus don't cause the spike in blood glucose levels that carbohydrates do. It is recommended that about half of your calories (from 45 to 65 percent) should come from carbohydrates.

Most people are much more likely to eat a meal that consists of a combination of carbohydrates, protein, and fat than a single nutrient alone. Therefore, paying attention to each of these elements within a meal will assist in blood glucose control. For example, when you eat a turkey sandwich, the protein from the turkey will delay the response that the carbohydrates in the bread would normally have on blood glucose levels if eaten alone. (To delay the response further, eat whole wheat bread, full of dietary fiber, which will leave you feeling full and satisfied until your next meal.)

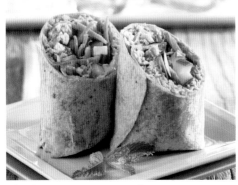

Chicken, Hummus and
Vegetable Wraps (page 88)

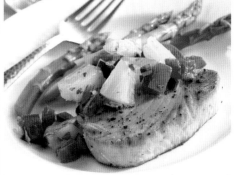

Tuna Steaks with Pineapple
and Tomato Salsa (page 134)

Portion Distortion

Regardless of what you're eating, one of the most important things that you should pay attention to is portion size. Learning to recognize all of the ingredients in a dish and the recommended serving sizes are fundamental tools to the success of any diet. Use the serving size listed on the Nutrition Facts panel on any packaged food or the nutrition information listed with the recipes in this book as a guide.

It is easy to get carried away, so always measure your portions—you'll be surprised how quickly they add up. Take breakfast cereals, for example. The serving size listed on the Nutrition Facts panel is 1 cup, but you probably pour more than that into your bowl. When you add the calories from the milk, you may be surprised at how many calories you're consuming.

Portion control is particularly crucial for people with diabetes in maintaining their blood glucose levels within a healthy range. Many people with diabetes will focus on their carbohydrate amounts and space their consumption throughout the day. This type of meal plan will help to prevent large spikes in blood glucose, as the goal for managing diabetes is to keep it at a steady, consistent level at all times.

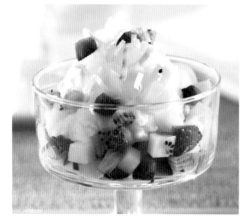 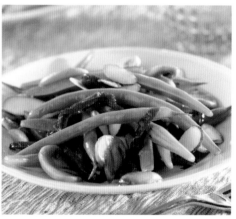

Toasted Coconut and
Tropical Fruit Parfaits (page 210)

Vegetables and Sun-Dried Tomatoes
(page 172)

Should You Use the Glycemic Index?

The glycemic index is a method for measuring whether an individual food causes an immediate surge in blood sugar (high glycemic foods) or a gradual rise in blood sugar (low glycemic foods). The idea behind the glycemic index is to allow you to compare the effect of various foods on your blood sugar and to make choices that help you maintain a more constant blood sugar. The glycemic index rates a food's capacity to raise blood sugar by comparing it to a standard—either white bread or glucose—that is given a rating of 100. If a food raises blood sugar faster than white bread, its rating is higher than 100. If it raises blood sugar more slowly than white bread, its rating will be lower.

If you're confused, don't worry—the glycemic index is actually even more complicated to use than it seems. That's because you rarely just eat carbohydrates. Meals and even individual foods may contain fat and fiber, both of which slow the breakdown of carbohydrate into glucose. A baked potato is a good example: Eat a plain one, and your blood sugar may soar. But if you add a pat of butter, it will rise more gradually. How much? That's hard to say. The cooking method, too, can affect how you metabolize a carbohydrate. For instance, pasta cooked al dente (firm) is absorbed more slowly than pasta that is cooked longer.

Furthermore, if you're sticking with healthy carbohydrate choices—that is, lots of fruits, vegetables and whole grains—you're probably eating at the low end of the glycemic index anyway. The American Diabetes Association has stated that while the glycemic index may be a useful tool in meal planning, the total amount of carbohydrates you consume is the most important factor in controlling blood sugar.

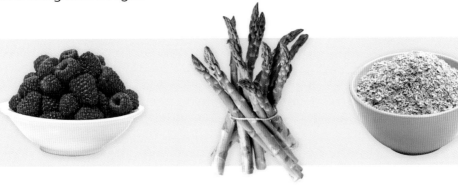

A Healthy Way of Life

What's the hot new weight-loss fad this year? Low-carb, high-protein, no-fat? Although fad diet books usually portray losing weight as a complicated process that requires following carefully prescribed steps, there is nothing mysterious about weight loss. You simply have to burn more calories than you eat.

But have you ever wondered what exactly a calorie is? Calories measure the amount of energy contained in a food or beverage; they also measure the amount of energy your body burns.

So does that mean that a 150-calorie can of soda is a better source of energy than a 6-calorie celery stalk? Not exactly. Unless you're very active, consuming a lot of high-calorie foods causes the body to store the unused fuel in the form of fat. To lose love handles and other unsightly fat deposits, you have to create a calorie deficit—that is, consume fewer than you burn. To drop one pound, you have to create a deficit of 3,500 calories.

However, as anyone who has ever gone on a weight-loss diet knows, the real challenge is keeping off the pounds. You will have a greater chance of success if you work with your registered dietitian to come up with a weight-loss plan that identifies which foods to eat, how many calories to consume each day and a reasonable target weight.

What is a Registered Dietitian?

Registered dietitians are nutrition experts who work in a variety of settings, including hospitals, clinics and private practices. A registered dietitian has to earn a bachelor's degree or higher from an accredited university or college and participate in a 6- to 12-month professional training program at a health care facility, community agency or food-service corporation. The candidate must then pass a certification exam. Some registered dietitians specialize in diabetes education. Your doctor or diabetes educator can recommend a registered dietitian to help you design a healthy meal plan. If you want to find one on your own, look for the credentials "R.D." after his or her name. A great place to start is the American Dietetic Association website.

Tips for Adding Veggies to Your Diet

1. Make it easy on yourself. When grocery shopping, choose prewashed bags of vegetables or bring home goodies from the salad bar.

2. Go vegetarian once a week. Plan a whole meal around a vegetable-based main dish. Try a soup, stew or pasta creation.

3. Cook with more veggies. Add veggies to your favorite dishes; try adding zucchini or carrots to meatloaves or breads.

4. Try something new and different. Add color and flavor to your menus with mustard greens, beets or different varieties of more common fruits and veggies such as Saturn peaches or Italian-style green beans.

5. Grow your own or shop locally. Grow vegetables in your garden or visit your local farmers' market or produce stand. You'll find different types of vegetables that will inspire you to cook.

6. Get colorful. Nutritionists believe that the same chemicals that give certain kinds of fruits and vegetables a brilliant hue may also promote health and help fight diseases. Tomatoes and watermelon, for instance, get their rich red color from an antioxidant called lycopene, which may prevent some cancers.

Get Cooking

This book is a guide and a resource for helping you create some of your favorite dishes and fit them into a healthy meal plan. The nutrition information with each recipe in this book is provided so that you'll be aware of how each dish will affect your blood glucose levels and fit within your diet. The nutrition information listed is based on a single serving and does not include garnishes or optional ingredients; when a range is given for an ingredient, the nutritional analysis reflects the lesser amount. Please consult a registered dietitian or health care provider who can offer nutrition advice, tips and meal plans that are all specific to you, your health condition and your lifestyle.

BREAKFAST

MEXICAN BREAKFAST BURRITO

1 container (16 ounces) cholesterol-free egg substitute
⅛ teaspoon black pepper
    Nonstick cooking spray
⅓ cup canned black beans, rinsed and drained
2 tablespoons sliced green onion
2 (10-inch) flour tortillas
3 tablespoons shredded reduced-fat Cheddar cheese
3 tablespoons salsa

1. Whisk egg substitute and pepper in medium bowl until well blended. Spray large nonstick skillet with cooking spray; heat over medium heat. Pour egg mixture into skillet; cook 5 to 7 minutes or until mixture begins to set, stirring occasionally. Stir in beans and green onion; cook and stir 3 minutes or just until cooked through.

2. Spoon mixture evenly down centers of tortillas; top evenly with cheese. Roll up to enclose filling. Cut in half; top with salsa.   *Makes 4 servings*

Nutrients per Serving: ½ *burrito*
Calories: 200, **Calories from Fat:** 18%, **Total Fat:** 4g,
Saturated Fat: 1g, **Cholesterol:** 5mg, **Sodium:** 590mg,
Carbohydrate: 22g, **Fiber:** 5g, **Protein:** 17g

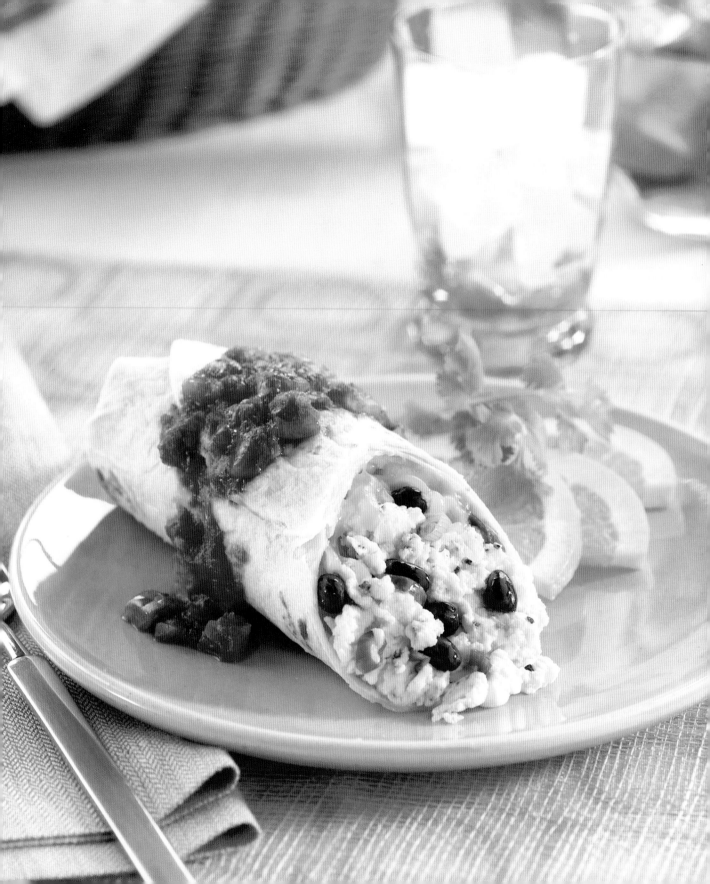

BERRY BRAN MUFFINS

    2 cups dry bran cereal
1¼ cups fat-free (skim) milk
  ½ cup packed brown sugar
  ¼ cup vegetable oil
  1 egg, lightly beaten
  1 teaspoon vanilla
1¼ cups all-purpose flour
  1 tablespoon baking powder
  ¼ teaspoon salt
  1 cup fresh or frozen blueberries, partially thawed

1. Preheat oven to 350°F. Line 12 standard (2½-inch) muffin cups with paper baking cups.

2. Combine cereal and milk in medium bowl. Let stand 5 minutes to soften. Add brown sugar, oil, egg and vanilla; beat well. Combine flour, baking powder and salt in large bowl. Stir in cereal mixture just until dry ingredients are moistened. Gently fold in blueberries. Spoon evenly into prepared muffin cups.

3. Bake 20 to 25 minutes for fresh blueberries or 25 to 30 minutes for frozen blueberries or until toothpick inserted into centers comes out clean. Serve warm.

Makes 12 muffins

Nutrients per Serving: *1 muffin*
Calories: 172, **Calories from Fat:** 27%, **Total Fat:** 5g,
Saturated Fat: 1g, **Cholesterol:** 18mg, **Sodium:** 287mg,
Carbohydrate: 29g, **Fiber:** 4g, **Protein:** 4g

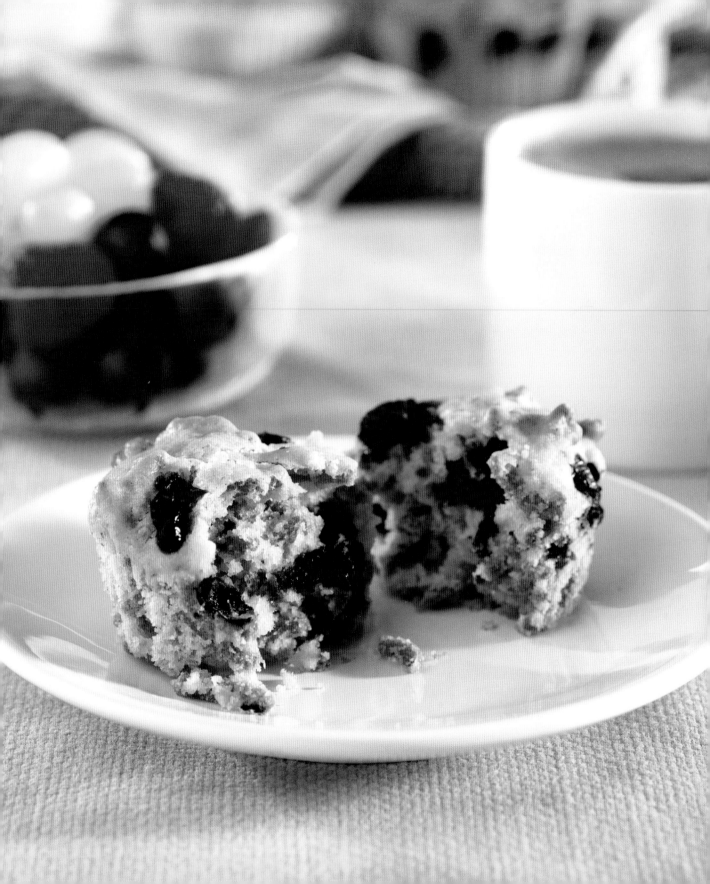

ASPARAGUS AND SCALLION OMELET WITH TORTILLA WEDGES

    8 ounces small asparagus spears, trimmed

    1 teaspoon olive oil

    ¼ teaspoon black pepper, divided

    5 egg whites

    ¼ cup shredded Parmesan cheese

    2 tablespoons minced green onion

    ⅛ teaspoon salt

       Dash chipotle chili powder

       Nonstick cooking spray

    1 (8-inch) whole wheat tortilla, warmed and cut into wedges*

Or you may substitute with 1 whole wheat pita bread round, cut in half.

1. Preheat oven to 425°F. Arrange asparagus on baking sheet; brush with oil and sprinkle with ⅛ teaspoon pepper. Roast 15 minutes or until asparagus are golden brown and tender. Cover and keep warm.

2. Beat egg whites in large bowl until foamy. Stir in cheese, green onion, salt remaining ⅛ teaspoon pepper and chili powder.

3. Spray large nonstick skillet with cooking spray; heat over medium-high heat. Pour egg white mixture into skillet; cook and stir gently, lifting edge to allow uncooked portion to flow underneath. Continue cooking until set.

4. Cut omelet in half and arrange each half on serving plate. Top each with half of asparagus. Serve each with half of tortilla wedges. *Makes 2 servings*

Nutrients per Serving: *½ of total recipe*
Calories: 152, **Calories from Fat:** 24%, **Total Fat:** 4g,
Saturated Fat: <1g, **Cholesterol:** 1mg, **Sodium:** 449mg,
Carbohydrate: 14g, **Fiber:** 2g, **Protein:** 15g

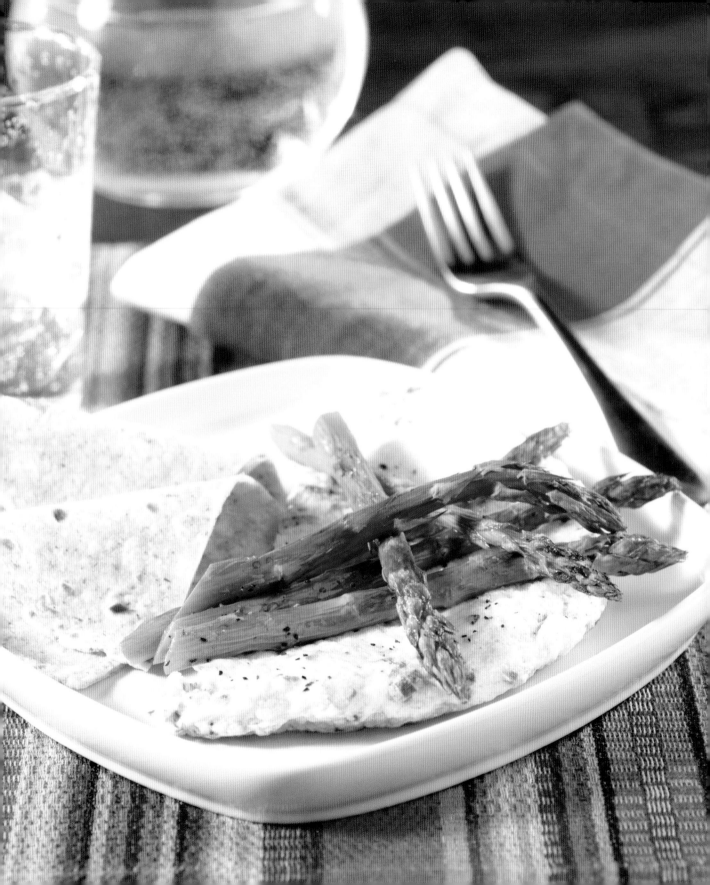

BUCKWHEAT PANCAKES

1 cup buckwheat flour
2 tablespoons cornstarch
2 teaspoons baking powder
¼ teaspoon salt
¼ teaspoon ground cinnamon
1 cup whole milk
1 egg
2 tablespoons butter, melted
2 tablespoons maple syrup
½ teaspoon vanilla
  Additional butter for cooking
  Additional maple syrup (optional)

1. Whisk buckwheat flour, cornstarch, baking powder, salt and cinnamon in medium bowl. Combine milk, egg, 2 tablespoons butter, 2 tablespoons maple syrup and vanilla in small bowl; whisk into dry ingredients just until combined. Let stand 5 minutes. (Batter will be thick and elastic.)

2. Heat additional butter in griddle or large nonstick skillet over medium heat. Pour ¼ cupfuls batter 2 inches apart onto griddle. Cook 2 minutes or until lightly browned and edges begin to bubble. Turn over; cook 2 minutes or until lightly browned. Repeat with remaining batter. Serve with additional maple syrup, if desired.

Makes 12 pancakes

Nutrients per Serving: *3 pancakes*
Calories: 251, **Calories from Fat:** 35%, **Total Fat:** 10g,
Saturated Fat: 5g, **Cholesterol:** 68mg, **Sodium:** 489mg,
Carbohydrate: 35g, **Fiber:** 3g, **Protein:** 7g

Variation: Add ½ cup blueberries to the batter.

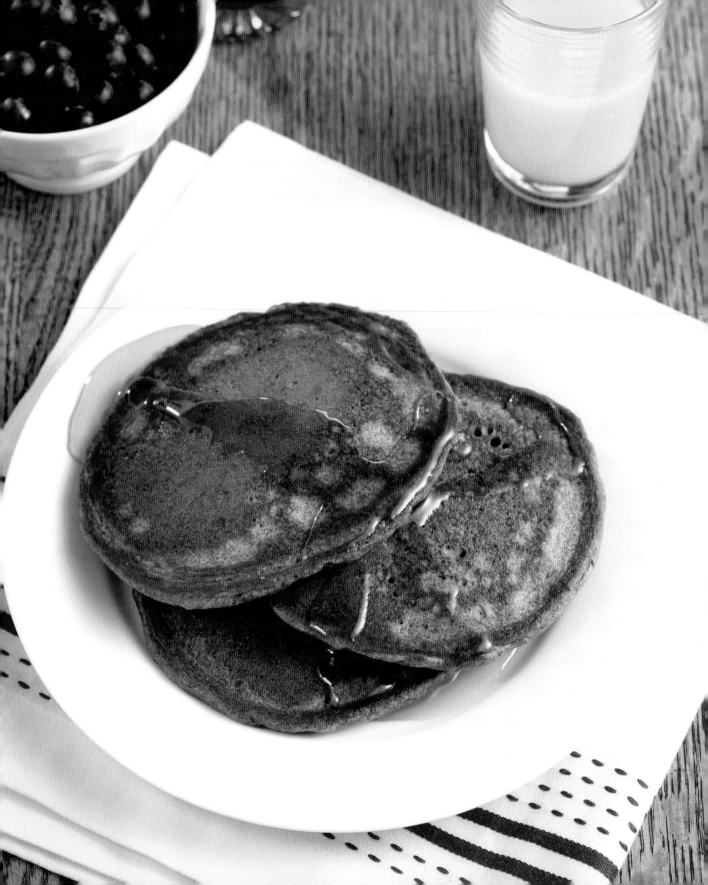

BREAKFAST PEPPERONI FLATS

    2 high-fiber low-fat flatbreads
    1 cup (4 ounces) shredded mozzarella cheese
    2 plum tomatoes, diced
   24 slices turkey pepperoni, cut into quarters
    2 teaspoons grated Parmesan cheese
   ¼ cup chopped fresh basil

1. Preheat oven to 425°F. Place flatbreads on baking sheet. Sprinkle evenly with mozzarella cheese, tomatoes, turkey pepperoni and Parmesan cheese.

2. Bake 3 minutes or until cheese is melted. Remove from oven. Sprinkle with basil. Let stand 2 minutes before slicing and serving.   *Makes 4 servings*

Nutrients per Serving: *¼ of total recipe*
Calories: 130, **Calories from Fat:** 28%, **Total Fat:** 4g,
Saturated Fat: 2g, **Cholesterol:** 20mg, **Sodium:** 520mg,
Carbohydrate: 9g, **Fiber:** 5g, **Protein:** 15g

TIP   To make this dish even more savory, top with additional veggies like mushrooms and onions.

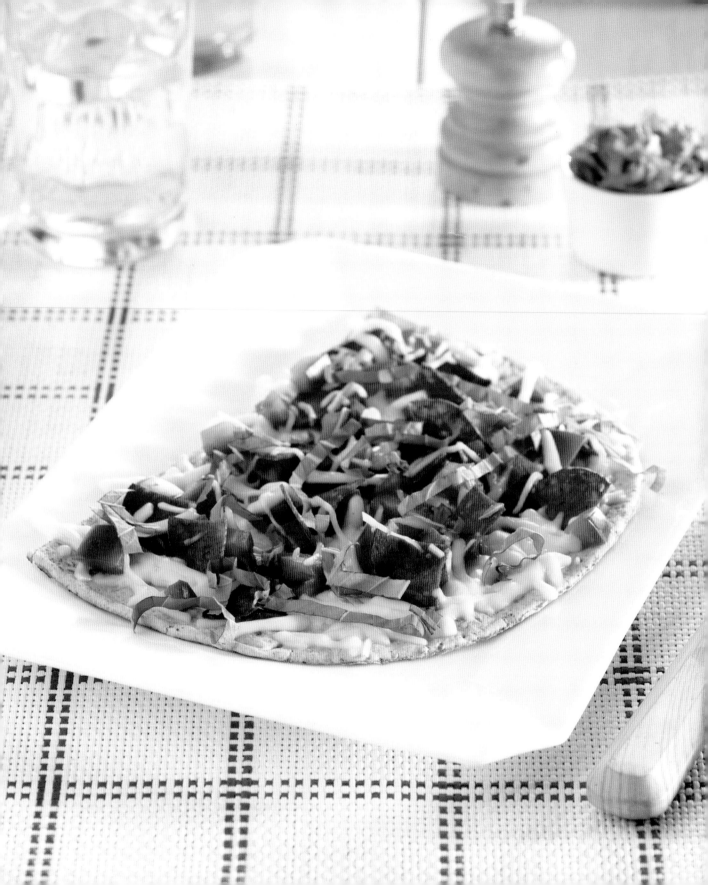

OATMEAL WITH MAPLE-GLAZED APPLES AND CRANBERRIES

3 cups water

¼ teaspoon salt

2 cups quick or old-fashioned oats

1 teaspoon unsalted butter

¼ teaspoon ground cinnamon

2 medium red or golden delicious apples, unpeeled, cut into ½-inch chunks

2 tablespoons sugar-free maple syrup

4 tablespoons dried cranberries

1. Bring water and salt to a boil in large saucepan. Stir in oats; reduce heat and simmer 1 to 2 minutes for quick oats or 5 to 6 minutes for old-fashioned oats.

2. Meanwhile, melt butter in large nonstick skillet over medium heat; stir in cinnamon. Add apples; cook and stir 4 to 5 minutes or until tender. Stir in maple syrup until heated through.

3. Spoon oatmeal evenly into four bowls; top evenly with apple mixture and cranberries.

Makes 4 servings

Nutrients per Serving: *¾ cup oatmeal with about ⅓ cup apple mixture and 1 tablespoon cranberries*
Calories: 230, **Calories from Fat:** 16%, **Total Fat:** 4g,
Saturated Fat: 1g, **Cholesterol:** 3mg, **Sodium:** 158mg,
Carbohydrate: 47g, **Fiber:** 6g, **Protein:** 6g

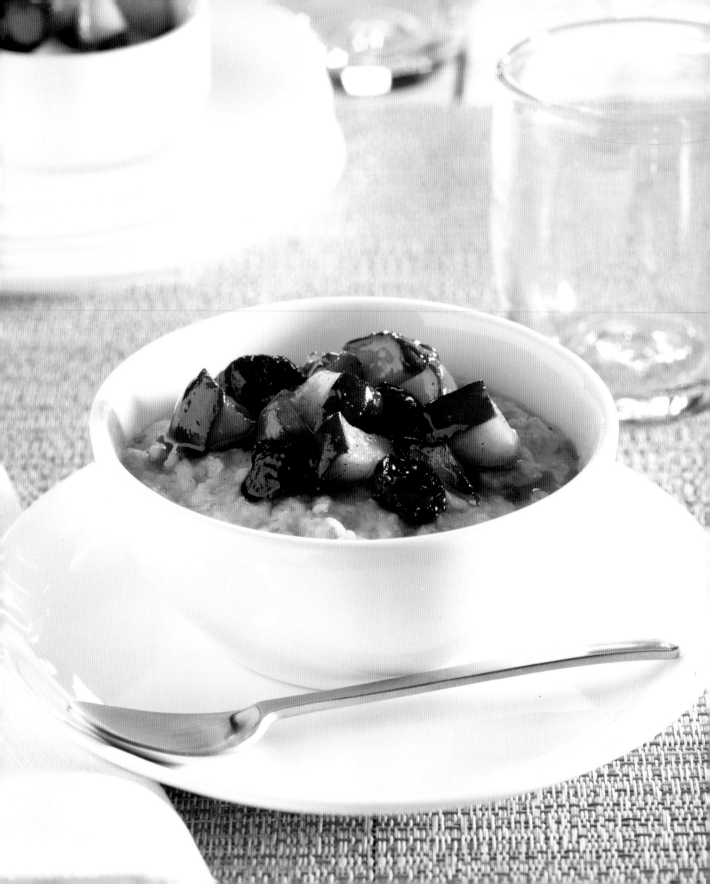

PEA AND SPINACH FRITTATA

Nonstick cooking spray
1 cup chopped onion
¼ cup water
1 cup frozen peas
1 cup torn stemmed spinach
6 egg whites
2 eggs
½ cup cooked brown rice
¼ cup fat-free (skim) milk
2 tablespoons grated Romano or Parmesan cheese, plus additional for garnish
1 tablespoon chopped fresh mint *or* 1 teaspoon dried mint leaves, crushed
¼ teaspoon black pepper
⅛ teaspoon salt

1. Spray large nonstick skillet with cooking spray. Combine onion and water in skillet; bring to a boil over high heat. Reduce heat to medium; cover and cook 2 to 3 minutes or until onion is tender. Stir in peas; cook until heated through. Drain. Add spinach; cook and stir 1 minute or until spinach just begins to wilt.

2. Whisk egg whites, eggs, rice, milk, 2 tablespoons cheese, mint, pepper and salt in medium bowl until well blended. Pour egg mixture into skillet; cook without stirring 2 minutes or until eggs begin to set. Gently lift edge to allow uncooked portion to flow underneath. Remove skillet from heat when eggs are almost set but surface is still moist. Cover; let stand 3 to 4 minutes or until surface is set.

3. To serve, cut into four wedges; sprinkle with additional cheese, if desired.

Makes 4 servings

Nutrients per Serving: *1 wedge*
Calories: 162, **Calories from Fat:** 22%, **Total Fat:** 4g,
Saturated Fat: 1g, **Cholesterol:** 110mg, **Sodium:** 246mg,
Carbohydrate: 18g, **Fiber:** 4g, **Protein:** 14g

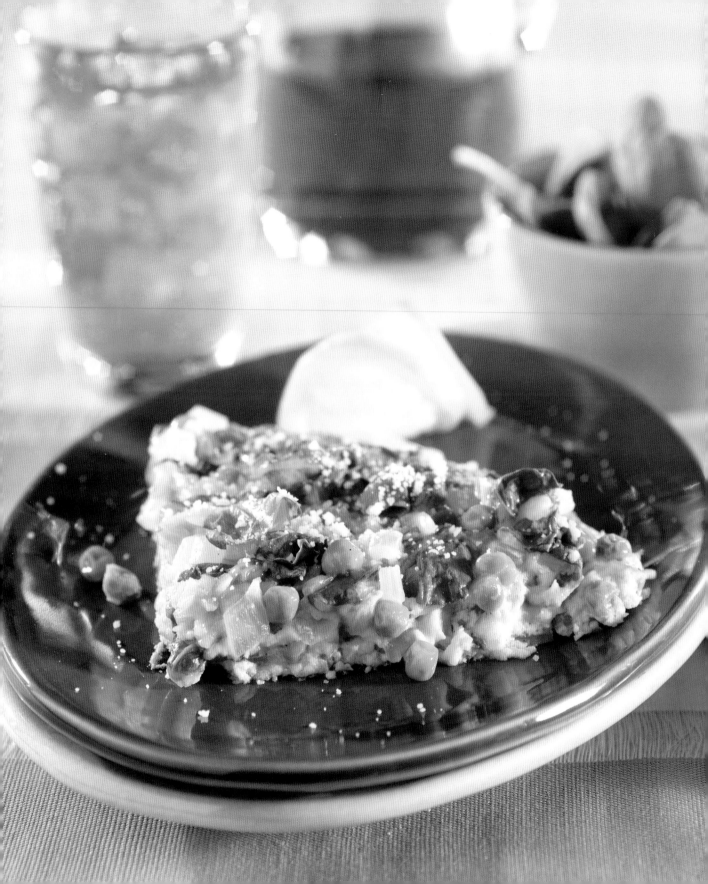

CINNAMON FRUIT CRUNCH

1 tablespoon butter

2 tablespoons plus 1 teaspoon packed brown sugar, divided

2¼ teaspoons ground cinnamon, divided

1 cup low-fat granola cereal

¼ cup sliced almonds, toasted*

½ cup vanilla nonfat yogurt

⅛ teaspoon ground nutmeg

2 cans (16 ounces each) mixed fruit chunks in juice, drained

To toast almonds, spread in single layer in heavy-bottomed skillet. Cook over medium heat 1 to 2 minutes, stirring frequently, until lightly browned. Remove from skillet immediately. Cool before using.

1. Melt butter in small saucepan over medium heat. Remove from heat; stir in 2 tablespoons brown sugar and 2 teaspoons cinnamon. Stir in granola and almonds; set aside to cool completely.

2. Stir yogurt, remaining 1 teaspoon brown sugar, ¼ teaspoon cinnamon and nutmeg in small bowl until well blended.

3. Spoon about ½ cup mixed fruit into each serving bowl. Top evenly with yogurt mixture; sprinkle evenly with granola mixture.   *Makes 6 servings*

Nutrients per Serving: *½ cup fruit with about 1 tablespoon yogurt mixture and 2 tablespoons granola mixture*
Calories: 259, **Calories from Fat:** 21%, **Total Fat:** 6g, **Saturated Fat:** 1g, **Cholesterol:** 1mg, **Sodium:** 109mg, **Carbohydrate:** 48g, **Fiber:** 6g, **Protein:** 4g

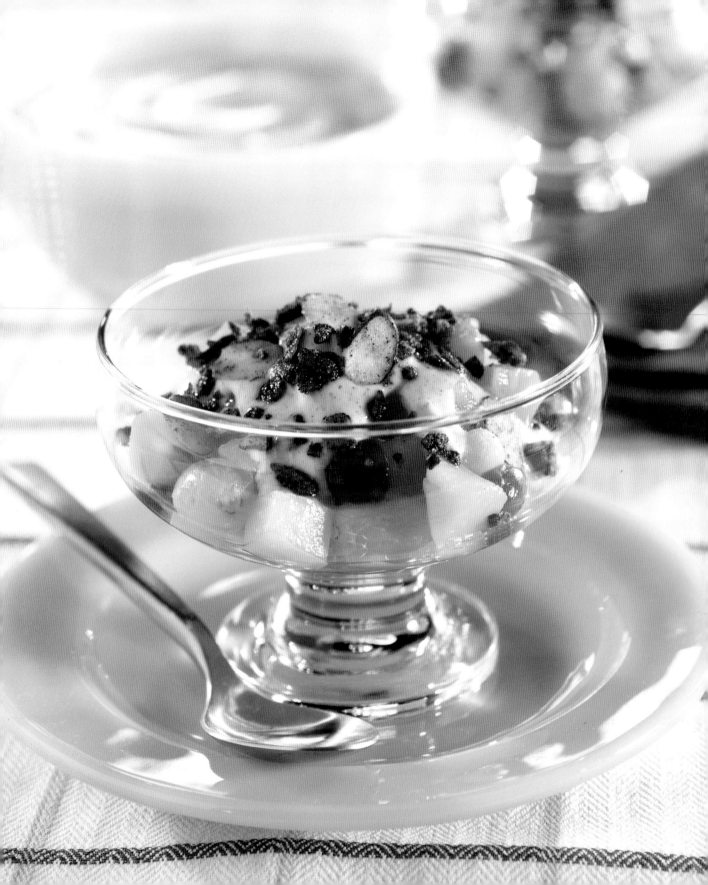

HAM & EGG BREAKFAST PANINI

  Nonstick cooking spray
¼ cup chopped green or red bell pepper
2 tablespoons sliced green onion
1 slice (1 ounce) reduced-fat smoked deli ham, chopped
½ cup cholesterol-free egg substitute
  Black pepper
4 slices multigrain or whole grain bread
2 slices (¾-ounce each) reduced-fat Cheddar or Swiss cheese

1. Spray small nonstick skillet with cooking spray; heat over medium heat. Add bell pepper and green onion; cook and stir 4 minutes or until crisp-tender. Stir in ham.

2. Whisk egg substitute and black pepper in small bowl until well blended. Pour egg mixture into skillet; cook 2 minutes or until egg mixture is almost set, stirring occasionally.

3. Heat grill pan or medium skillet over medium heat. Spray one side of each bread slice with cooking spray; turn bread over. Top each bread slice with 1 cheese slice and half of egg mixture. Top with second bread slice. Repeat with remaining bread slices, cheese slices and egg mixture.

4. Grill 2 minutes per side, pressing down lightly with spatula until toasted. (Cover pan with lid during last 2 minutes of cooking to melt cheese, if desired.) Serve immediately.

Makes 2 paninis

Nutrients per Serving: *1 panini*
Calories: 271, **Calories from Fat:** 17%, **Total Fat:** 5g,
Saturated Fat: 1g, **Cholesterol:** 9mg, **Sodium:** 577mg,
Carbohydrate: 30g, **Fiber:** 6g, **Protein:** 24g

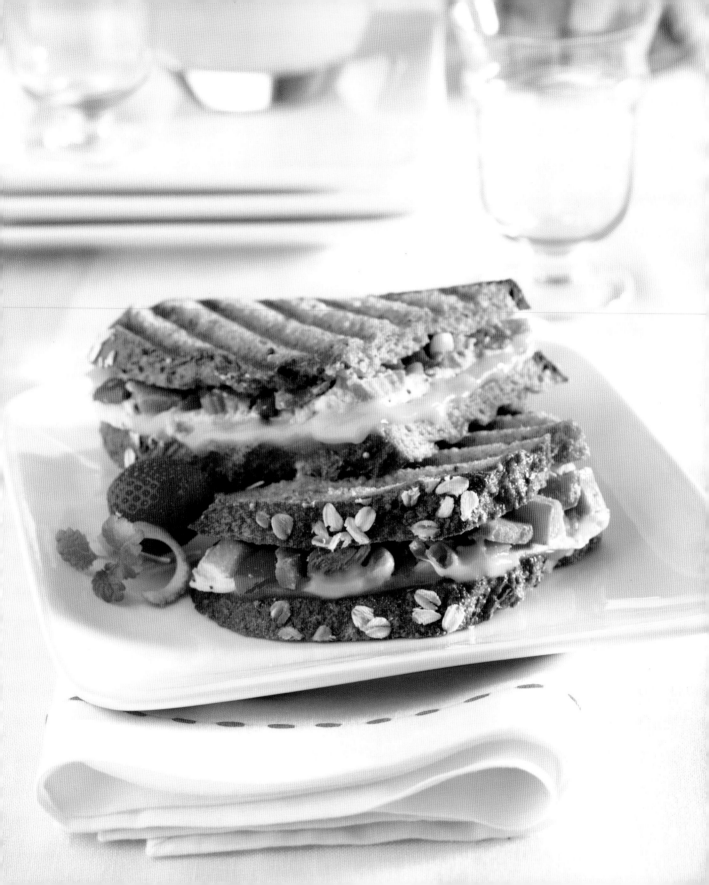

BRUNCH TIME ZUCCHINI-DATE BREAD

Bread

- 1 cup chopped pitted dates
- 1 cup water
- 1 cup whole wheat flour
- 1 cup all-purpose flour
- 2 tablespoons granulated sugar
- 1 teaspoon baking powder
- ½ teaspoon baking soda
- ½ teaspoon salt
- ½ teaspoon ground cinnamon
- ¼ teaspoon ground cloves
- 2 eggs
- 1 cup shredded zucchini, pressed dry with paper towels

Cream Cheese Spread

- 1 package (8 ounces) fat-free cream cheese
- ¼ cup powdered sugar
- 1 tablespoon vanilla
- ⅛ teaspoon ground cinnamon
- Dash ground cloves

1. Preheat oven to 350°F. Spray 8×4-inch loaf pan with nonstick cooking spray.

2. Combine dates and water in small saucepan; bring to a boil over medium-high heat. Remove from heat; let stand 15 minutes.

3. Combine flours, granulated sugar, baking powder, baking soda, salt, ½ teaspoon cinnamon and ¼ teaspoon cloves in large bowl. Beat eggs in medium bowl; stir in date mixture and zucchini. Stir egg mixture into flour mixture just until moistened. Pour into prepared pan.

continued on page 44

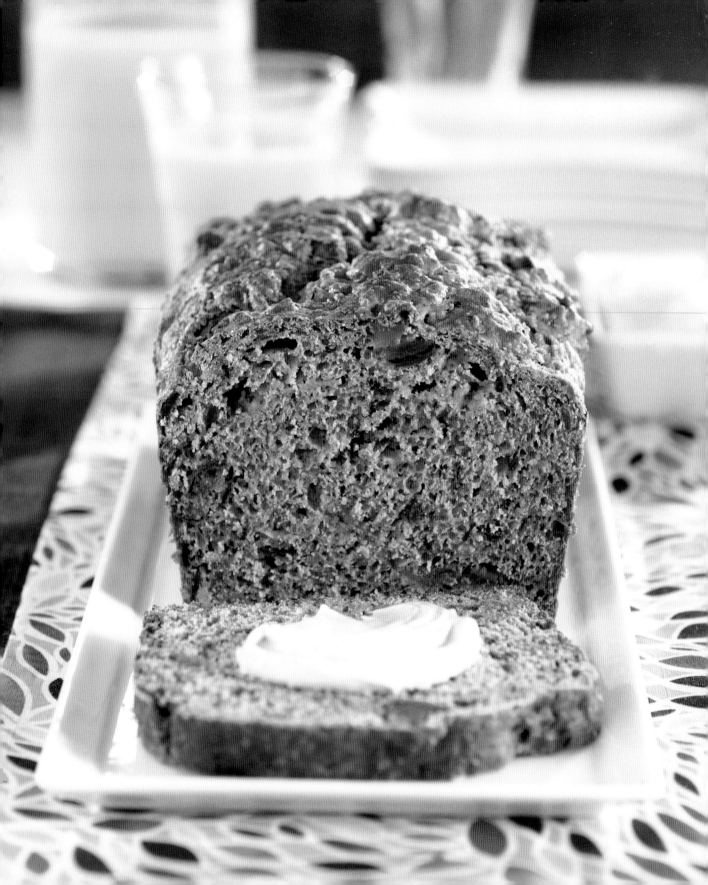

Brunch Time Zucchini-Date Bread, continued

4. Bake 30 to 35 minutes or until toothpick inserted into center comes out clean. Cool 5 minutes. Remove to wire rack; cool completely.

5. Meanwhile, prepare Cream Cheese Spread. Beat cream cheese, powdered sugar, vanilla, ⅛ teaspoon cinnamon and dash cloves in small bowl until smooth and well blended. Cover and refrigerate until ready to serve.

6. Cut bread into 16 slices. Serve with Cream Cheese Spread.   *Makes 16 servings*

Nutrients per Serving: *1 slice with about 1 tablespoon spread*
Calories: 124, **Calories from Fat:** 7%, **Total Fat:** 1g,
Saturated Fat: <1g, **Cholesterol:** 27mg, **Sodium:** 260mg,
Carbohydrate: 24g, **Fiber:** 2g, **Protein:** 5g

WHOA BREAKFAST

    3 cups water
    2 cups chopped peeled apples
  1½ cups steel-cut or old-fashioned oats
    ¼ cup sliced almonds
    ½ teaspoon ground cinnamon

Slow Cooker Directions

Combine water, apples, oats, almonds and cinnamon in slow cooker. Cover; cook on LOW 8 hours.   *Makes 6 servings*

Nutrients per Serving: *½ cup*
Calories: 119, **Calories from Fat:** 24%, **Total Fat:** 3g,
Saturated Fat: <1g, **Cholesterol:** 0mg, **Sodium:** <1mg,
Carbohydrate: 20g, **Fiber:** 4g, **Protein:** 3g

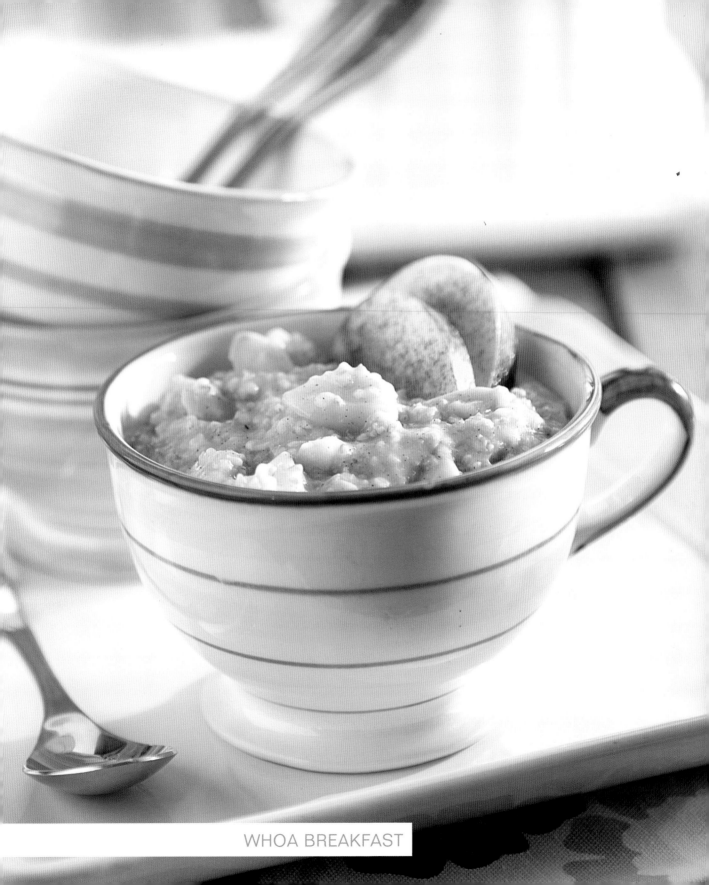

WHOA BREAKFAST

GREEN PEPPER SAUSAGE GRITS

1½ cups water

½ cup quick-cooking grits

Nonstick cooking spray

6 ounces turkey breakfast sausage links, removed from casings

1 cup diced green bell pepper

2 cloves garlic, minced

1 cup grape tomatoes, quartered

¼ cup water

¼ cup finely chopped green onions

2 teaspoons extra virgin olive oil

⅛ teaspoon ground red pepper

¼ teaspoon salt, divided

2 tablespoons chopped fresh parsley

1. Bring water to a boil in medium saucepan over high heat; stir in grits. Reduce heat to low; cover and simmer 6 minutes or until thickened.

2. Meanwhile, spray large nonstick skillet with cooking spray; heat over medium-high heat. Add sausage; cook 5 minutes or until browned, stirring frequently to break up meat. Remove to plate; set aside.

3. Spray same skillet with cooking spray. Add bell pepper; cook and stir 3 minutes. Stir in garlic. Add tomatoes; cook 3 minutes or until softened. Stir in water until well blended. Remove from heat. Stir sausage and any accumulated juices, green onions, oil, ground red pepper and ⅛ teaspoon salt into skillet; heat through.

4. Stir remaining ⅛ teaspoon salt into grits. Divide evenly among four bowls; spoon sausage mixture evenly over grits. Sprinkle evenly with parsley.   *Makes 4 servings*

Nutrients per Serving: *¼ of total recipe*
Calories: 210, **Calories from Fat:** 43%, **Total Fat:** 10g,
Saturated Fat: 3g, **Cholesterol:** 26mg, **Sodium:** 545mg,
Carbohydrate: 21g, **Fiber:** 2g, **Protein:** 9g

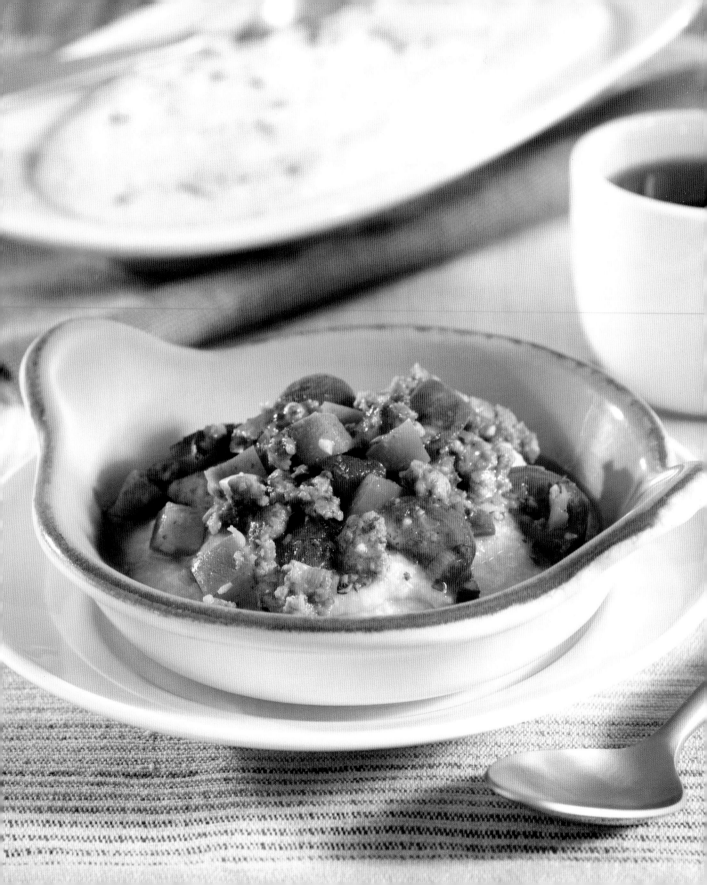

WHOLE GRAIN FRENCH TOAST

½ cup cholesterol-free egg substitute *or* 2 egg whites
¼ cup low-fat (1%) milk
½ teaspoon ground cinnamon
¼ teaspoon ground nutmeg
4 teaspoons butter
8 slices 100% whole wheat or multigrain bread
⅓ cup pure maple syrup
1 cup fresh blueberries
2 teaspoons powdered sugar

1. Preheat oven to 400°F. Spray baking sheet with nonstick cooking spray.

2. Whisk egg substitute, milk, cinnamon and nutmeg in shallow bowl until well blended. Melt 1 teaspoon butter in large nonstick skillet over medium heat. Working with two slices at a time, dip each bread slice in milk mixture, turning to coat both sides; let excess mixture drip back into bowl. Cook 2 minutes per side or until golden brown. Transfer to prepared baking sheet. Repeat with remaining butter, bread slices and milk mixture.

3. Bake 5 to 6 minutes or until heated through.

4. Meanwhile, microwave syrup in small microwavable bowl on HIGH 30 seconds or until bubbly. Stir in blueberries.

5. Divide French toast among four serving plates; top evenly with blueberry mixture. Sprinkle evenly with powdered sugar.
Makes 4 serving

Nutrients per Serving: *2 slices French toast with about ¼ cup blueberry mixture*
Calories: 251, **Calories from Fat:** 22%, **Total Fat:** 6g, **Saturated Fat:** 3g, **Cholesterol:** 11mg, **Sodium:** 324mg, **Carbohydrate:** 46g, **Fiber:** 5g, **Protein:** 12g

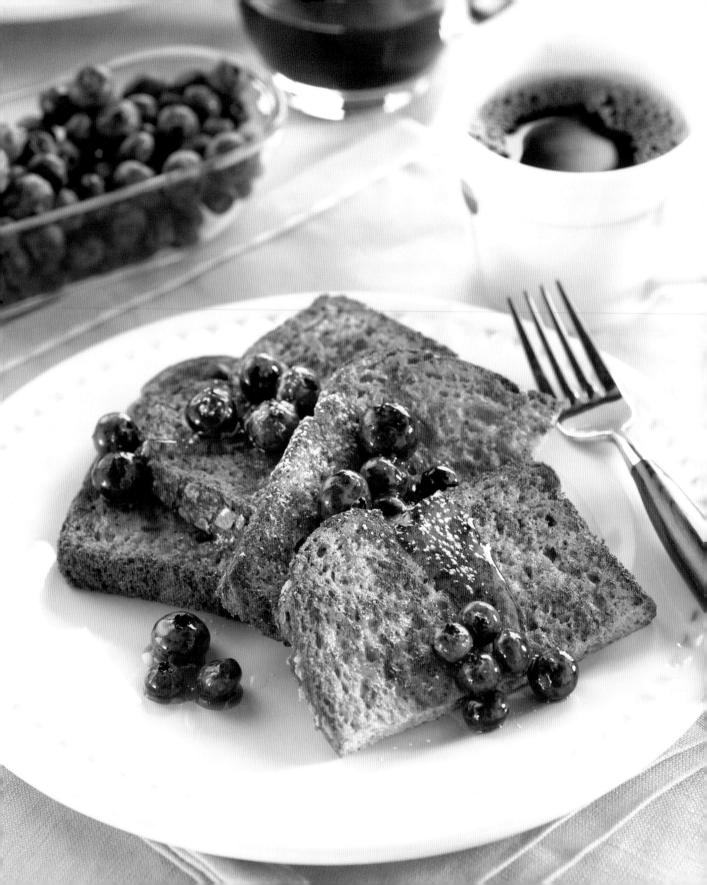

SCRAMBLED EGG AND RED PEPPER POCKETS

    1 egg
    2 egg whites
    1 tablespoon fat-free (skim) milk
  ⅛ teaspoon salt (optional)
  ⅛ teaspoon black pepper
1½ teaspoons unsalted butter, softened and divided
    3 tablespoons minced red onion
    2 tablespoons diced jarred roasted red pepper
    1 whole wheat pita bread round, cut in half crosswise

1. Whisk egg, egg whites, milk, salt, if desired, and black pepper in small bowl until well blended.

2. Melt ½ teaspoon butter in medium skillet over medium heat. Add onion; cook and stir 3 to 5 minutes or until lightly browned. Pour egg mixture into skillet; sprinkle with red pepper. Stir gently, lifting edge to allow uncooked portion to flow underneath. Continue cooking until set.

3. Evenly spread inside of each pita half with remaining 1 teaspoon butter. Spoon egg mixture into pita halves. *Makes 2 servings*

Nutrients per Serving: *1 pita half*
Calories: 155, **Calories from Fat:** 35%, **Total Fat:** 6g,
Saturated Fat: 3g, **Cholesterol:** 113mg, **Sodium:** 285mg,
Carbohydrate: 17g, **Fiber:** 3g, **Protein:** 8g

Note: An ideal breakfast includes lean protein, complex carbohydrates and a little bit of fat. This recipe includes all of the important aspects for a nutritious meal; it's filling enough to get you through the morning.

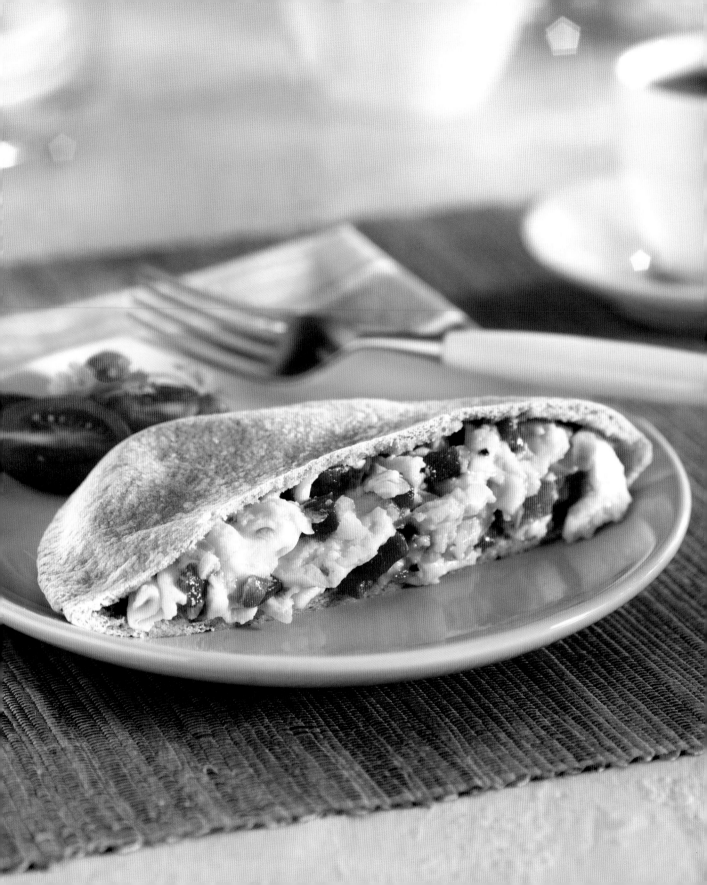

WHOLE WHEAT PUMPKIN MUFFINS

1½ cups whole wheat flour

¼ cup sugar

1 teaspoon salt

1 teaspoon ground allspice

1 teaspoon ground nutmeg

¾ teaspoon baking powder

½ teaspoon baking soda

¾ cup canned pumpkin

½ cup canola oil

½ cup honey

½ cup frozen apple juice concentrate, thawed

½ cup chopped walnuts

½ cup golden raisins

1. Preheat oven to 350°F. Spray 12 standard (2½-inch) muffin cups with nonstick cooking spray.

2. Combine flour, sugar, salt, allspice, nutmeg, baking powder and baking soda in large bowl; mix well. Stir in pumpkin, oil, honey and apple juice concentrate until well blended. Stir in walnuts and raisins. Spoon evenly into prepared muffin cups.

3. Bake 12 to 15 minutes or until toothpick inserted into centers comes out clean. Remove to wire rack; cool completely. *Makes 12 muffins*

Nutrients per Serving: *1 muffin*
Calories: 268, **Calories from Fat:** 40%, **Total Fat:** 12g,
Saturated Fat: 1g, **Cholesterol:** 0mg, **Sodium:** 283mg,
Carbohydrate: 39g, **Fiber:** 3g, **Protein:** 3g

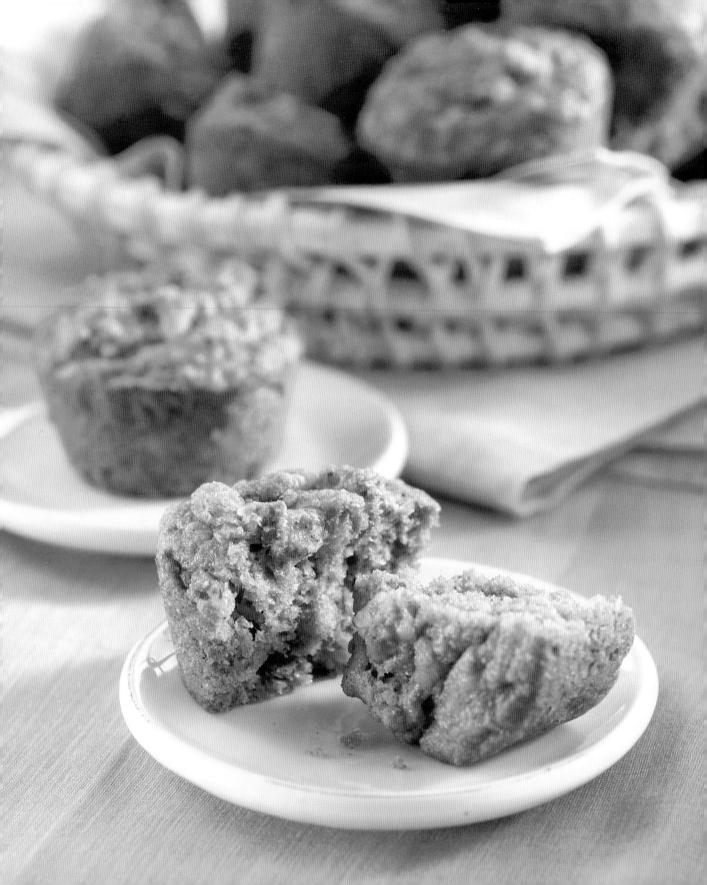

OATMEAL BANANA PANCAKES

1⅓ cups fat-free (skim) milk
½ cup quick oats
1 cup all-purpose flour
2 teaspoons baking powder
1 egg, lightly beaten
2 teaspoons canola oil
1 large banana, peeled and mashed
Nonstick cooking spray
½ cup sugar-free strawberry preserves

1. Combine milk and oats in large bowl; let stand 10 minutes.

2. Sift flour and baking powder into medium bowl. Stir flour mixture, egg and oil into oat mixture until moistened. Stir in banana.

3. Spray large griddle or skillet with cooking spray; heat over medium heat. Pour ¼ cupfuls batter 2 inches apart onto griddle; cook 2 to 3 minutes or until tops bubble and bottoms are golden brown. Turn over; cook 1 to 2 minutes or until golden brown.

4. Microwave preserves in small microwavable bowl on HIGH 1 minute or until heated through.

5. Place 3 pancakes on each serving plate; top with 2 tablespoons preserves.

Makes 6 servings

Nutrients per Serving: *3 pancakes with about 2 tablespoons preserves*
Calories: 176, **Calories from Fat:** 15%, **Total Fat:** 3g,
Saturated Fat: 1g, **Cholesterol:** 36mg, **Sodium:** 198mg,
Carbohydrate: 35g, **Fiber:** 2g, **Protein:** 6g

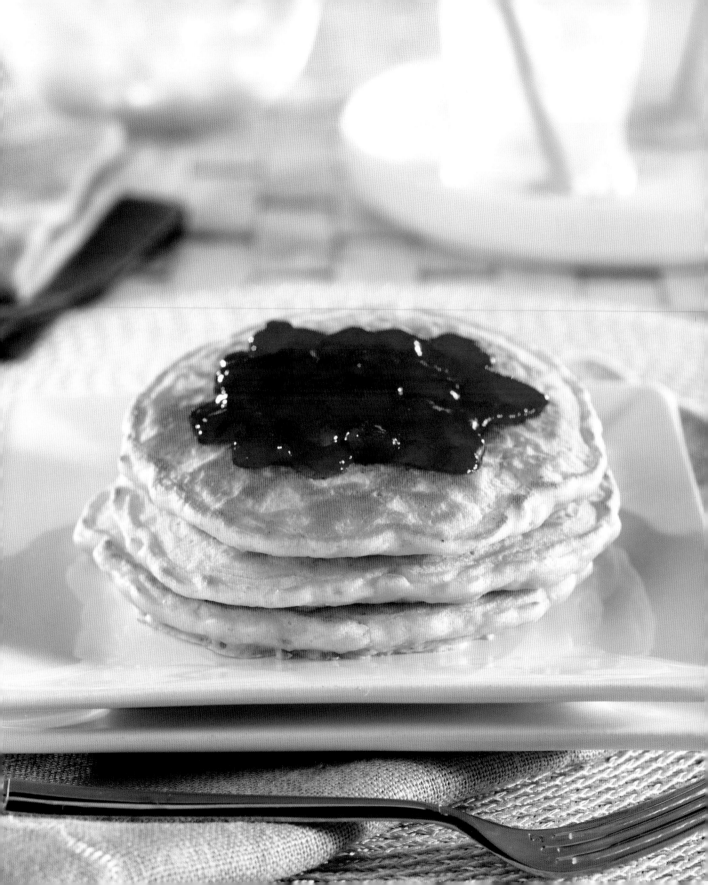

SALADS & SOUPS

TOMATO, AVOCADO AND CUCUMBER SALAD WITH FETA CHEESE

1½ tablespoons extra virgin olive oil

1 tablespoon balsamic vinegar

1 clove garlic, minced

¼ teaspoon salt

¼ teaspoon black pepper

2 cups diced seeded plum tomatoes

1 small ripe avocado, peeled, seeded and diced

½ cup chopped cucumber

⅓ cup crumbled reduced-fat feta cheese

4 large red leaf lettuce leaves

Chopped fresh basil (optional)

Whisk oil, vinegar, garlic, salt and pepper in medium bowl. Add tomatoes and avocado; toss to coat. Stir in cucumber and cheese. Arrange lettuce on serving plates. Spoon salad evenly onto lettuce. Garnish with basil. *Makes 4 servings*

Nutrients per Serving: ¼ *of total recipe*
Calories: 138, **Calories from Fat:** 72%, **Total Fat:** 11g,
Saturated Fat: 2g, **Cholesterol:** 3mg, **Sodium:** 311mg,
Carbohydrate: 7g, **Fiber:** 2g, **Protein:** 4g

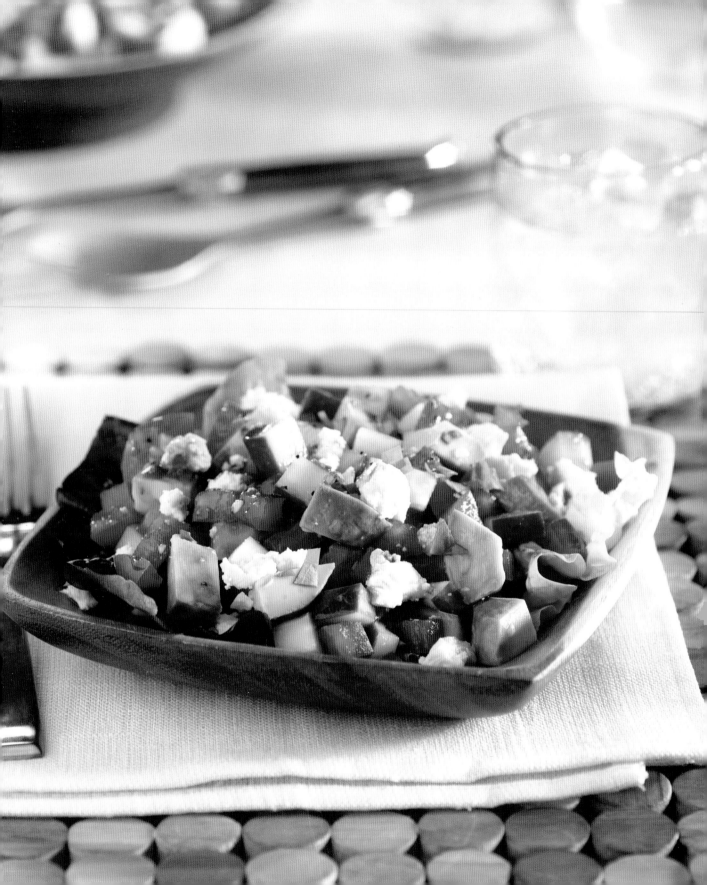

MINESTRONE ALLA MILANESE

2 cans (about 14 ounces each) reduced-sodium beef broth
1 can (about 14 ounces) diced tomatoes, undrained
1 cup diced potato
1 cup coarsely chopped carrots
1 cup coarsely chopped green cabbage
1 cup sliced zucchini
¾ cup chopped onion
¾ cup sliced fresh green beans
¾ cup coarsely chopped celery
¾ cup water
2 tablespoons olive oil
1 clove garlic, minced
½ teaspoon dried basil
¼ teaspoon dried rosemary
1 bay leaf
1 can (about 15 ounces) cannellini beans, rinsed and drained
Shredded Parmesan cheese (optional)

Slow Cooker Directions

1. Combine all ingredients except cannellini beans and cheese in 5-quart slow cooker; mix well. Cover; cook on LOW 5 to 6 hours.

2. Add cannellini beans. Cover; cook on LOW 1 hour or until vegetables are tender.

3. Remove and discard bay leaf. Ladle soup into bowls; garnish with cheese.

Makes 8 servings

Nutrients per Serving: *1½ cups*
Calories: 135, **Calories from Fat:** 27%, **Total Fat:** 4g,
Saturated Fat: 1g, **Cholesterol:** 0mg, **Sodium:** 242mg,
Carbohydrate: 23g, **Fiber:** 5g, **Protein:** 8g

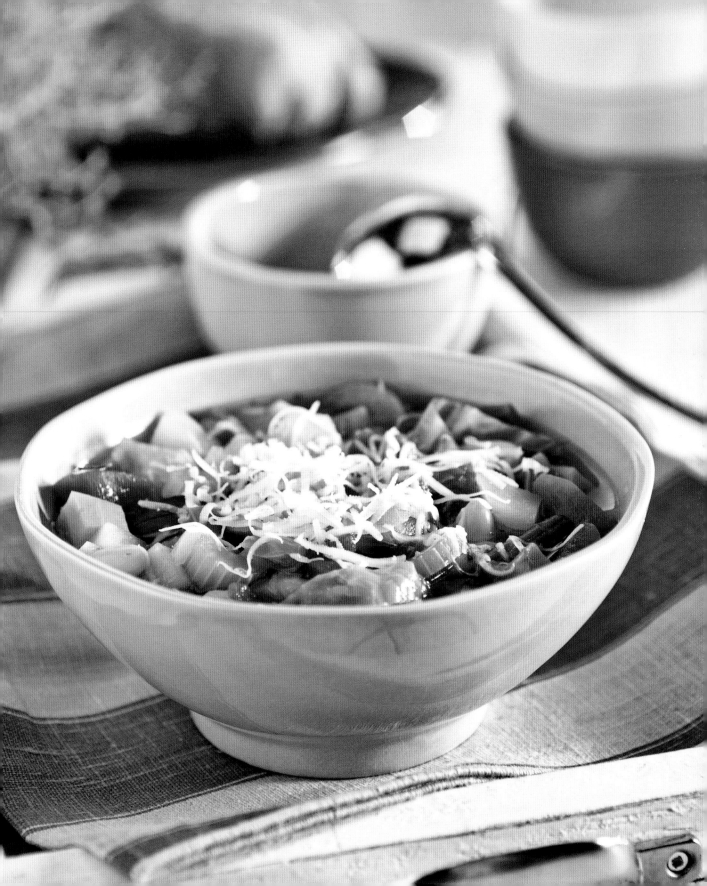

STRAWBERRY SPINACH SALAD WITH POPPY SEED DRESSING

2 tablespoons canola oil

2 tablespoons unseasoned rice or raspberry vinegar

2 teaspoons honey

1 teaspoon ground dry mustard

   Black pepper

½ teaspoon poppy seeds

6 cups baby spinach

8 strawberries, halved

½ ounce pecans, chopped and toasted*

¼ cup sliced red onion

1½ ounces goat cheese, broken into small pieces

To toast pecans, spread in single layer in heavy-bottomed skillet. Cook over medium heat 1 to 2 minutes, stirring frequently, until lightly browned. Remove from skillet immediately. Cool before using.

1. Whisk oil, vinegar, honey, mustard, pepper and poppy seeds in small bowl until well blended; set aside.

2. Arrange spinach evenly on four serving plates. Top evenly with strawberries, pecans, onion and cheese. Drizzle evenly with dressing.   *Makes 4 servings*

Nutrients per Serving: *1½ cups salad with about ½ tablespoon dressing*
Calories: 164, **Calories from Fat:** 66%, **Total Fat:** 12g, **Saturated Fat:** 2g, **Cholesterol:** 5mg, **Sodium:** 98mg, **Carbohydrate:** 11g, **Fiber:** 3g, **Protein:** 4g

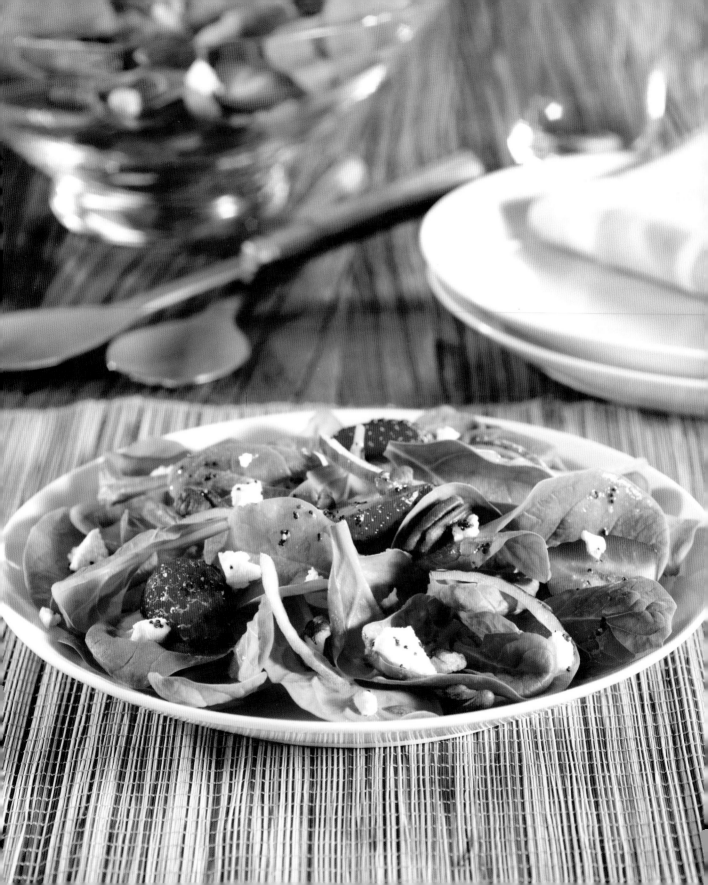

TANGY VEGETABLE SALAD

2 cups small broccoli florets
1 cup finely shredded red cabbage
¾ cup diced red bell pepper
1 medium carrot, shredded (about ½ cup)
½ cup fat-free or reduced-fat ranch salad dressing
2 teaspoons prepared horseradish

Combine broccoli, cabbage, bell pepper and carrot in large bowl. Whisk salad dressing and horseradish in small bowl until well blended. Pour over vegetables; toss to coat. Cover and refrigerate until ready to serve.   *Makes 6 servings*

Nutrients per Serving: *½ cup*
Calories: 56, **Calories from Fat:** 8%, **Total Fat:** 1g,
Saturated Fat: <1g, **Cholesterol:** 1mg, **Sodium:** 225mg,
Carbohydrate: 11g, **Fiber:** 2g, **Protein:** 2g

TIP   This salad is as versatile as it is easy to make. It can be prepared a day ahead and served warm or cold—perfect for potlucks, picnics and even lunch boxes.

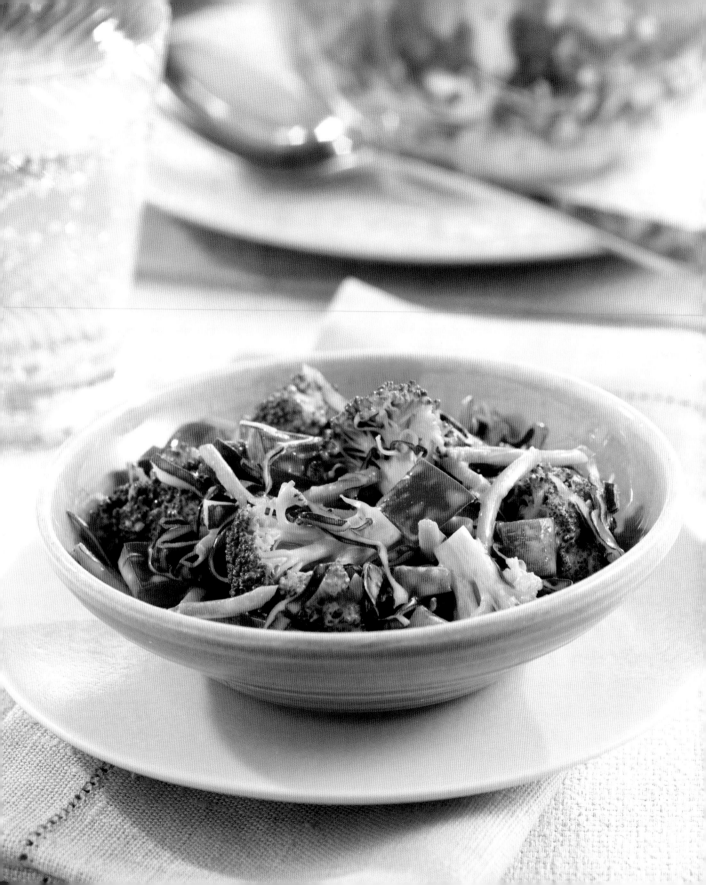

ONION SOUP WITH PASTA

    Nonstick cooking spray

3 cups sliced onions

3 cloves garlic, minced

½ teaspoon sugar

2 cans (about 14 ounces each) reduced-sodium beef broth

½ cup uncooked small bowtie pasta

2 tablespoons dry sherry

¼ teaspoon salt

⅛ teaspoon black pepper

    Grated Parmesan cheese (optional)

1. Spray large saucepan with cooking spray; heat over medium heat. Add onions and garlic; cover and cook 5 to 8 minutes or until onions are softened. Stir in sugar; cook 15 minutes or until onion mixture is very soft and browned.

2. Pour broth into saucepan; bring to a boil. Add pasta and simmer, uncovered, 6 to 8 minutes or until tender. Stir in sherry, salt and pepper. Ladle soup into bowls; garnish with cheese.

Makes 4 servings

Nutrients per Serving: *¼ of total recipe*
Calories: 141, **Calories from Fat:** 3%, **Total Fat:** 1g,
Saturated Fat: <1g, **Cholesterol:** 0mg, **Sodium:** 201mg,
Carbohydrate: 25g, **Fiber:** 2g, **Protein:** 8g

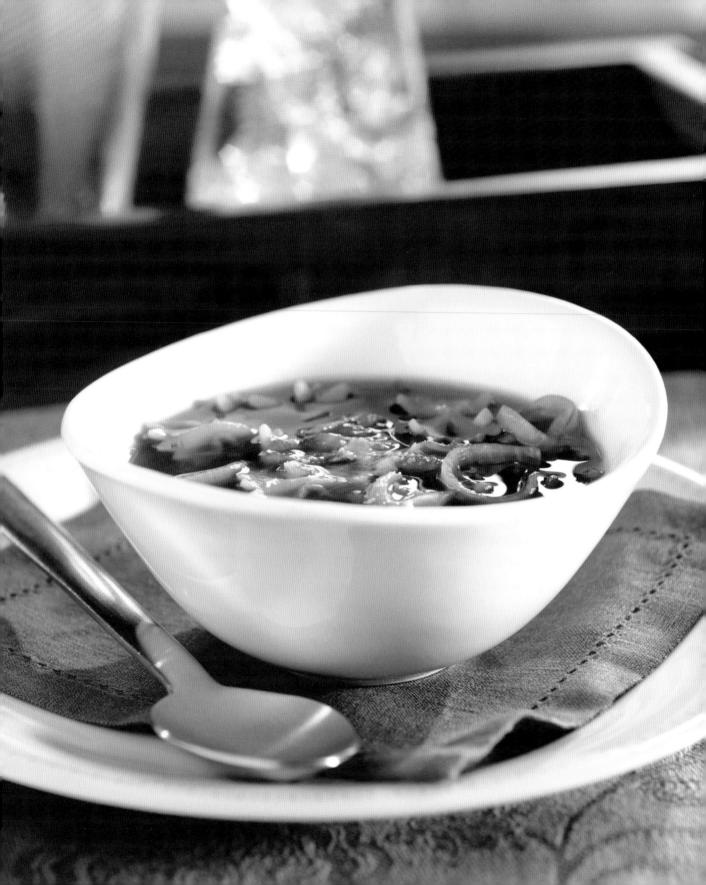

MARINATED TOMATO SALAD

1½ cups white wine or tarragon vinegar

½ teaspoon salt

¼ cup finely chopped shallots

2 tablespoons finely chopped chives

2 tablespoons fresh lemon juice

¼ teaspoon ground white pepper

2 tablespoons extra virgin olive oil

6 plum tomatoes, quartered

2 large yellow tomatoes,* sliced horizontally into ½-inch thick slices

16 red cherry tomatoes, halved

16 small yellow pear tomatoes,* halved (optional)

Sunflower sprouts (optional)

*You may substitute 10 plum tomatoes, quartered, for the yellow tomatoes.

1. Combine vinegar and salt in large bowl; stir until salt is completely dissolved. Add shallots, chives, lemon juice and white pepper; mix well. Slowly whisk in oil until well blended.

2. Add tomatoes to marinade; toss well. Cover; let stand at room temperature 30 minutes or up to 2 hours before serving.

3. To serve, divide salad evenly among eight serving plates. Top with sunflower sprouts, if desired.   *Makes 8 servings*

Nutrients per Serving: *1¼ cups*
Calories: 72, **Calories from Fat:** 45%, **Total Fat:** 4g,
Saturated Fat: <1g, **Cholesterol:** 0mg, **Sodium:** 163mg,
Carbohydrate: 9g, **Fiber:** 2g, **Protein:** 2g

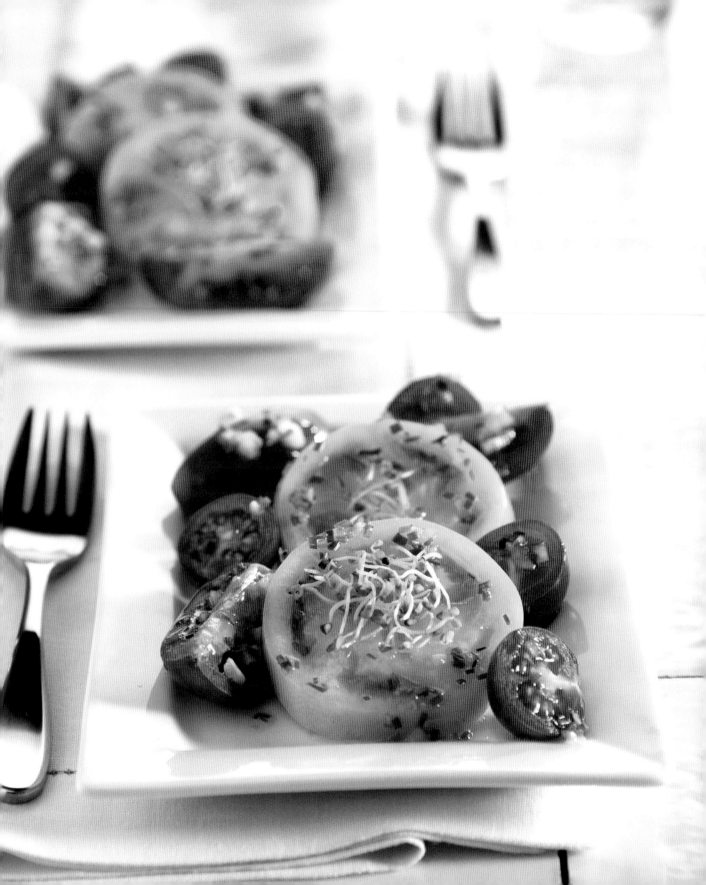

VEGETABLE LENTIL SOUP WITH CILANTRO

    Nonstick cooking spray
 2 medium carrots, thinly sliced
 ½ cup chopped onion
 4 cups water
 ¾ cup dried lentils, rinsed and sorted*
 2 teaspoons chicken bouillon or vegetarian chicken-flavored bouillon
 ½ teaspoon ground cumin
 ⅛ teaspoon ground red pepper
 1 medium tomato, diced
 ½ cup chopped roasted red bell peppers
 2 teaspoons olive oil
 ¼ teaspoon salt (optional)
 2 tablespoons chopped fresh cilantro

Packages of dried lentils may contain grits and tiny stones. Thoroughly rinse lentils then sort through them and discard any unusual looking pieces.

1. Spray large saucepan or Dutch oven with cooking spray; heat over medium-high heat. Add carrots and onion; cook and stir 4 minutes or until onion is translucent.

2. Add water, lentils, bouillon, cumin and ground red pepper. Bring to a boil over high heat. Reduce heat; cover and simmer 45 minutes or until lentils are very tender.

3. Remove from heat; stir in tomato, roasted red peppers, oil and salt, if desired. Cover and let stand 5 minutes before serving. Ladle soup into bowls; garnish with cilantro.

Makes 4 servings

Nutrients per Serving: *1 cup*
Calories: 182, **Calories from Fat:** 14%, **Total Fat:** 3g,
Saturated Fat: 1g, **Cholesterol:** 0mg, **Sodium:** 466mg,
Carbohydrate: 29g, **Fiber:** 13g, **Protein:** 11g

Note: This soup keeps well and is even more flavorful the next day.

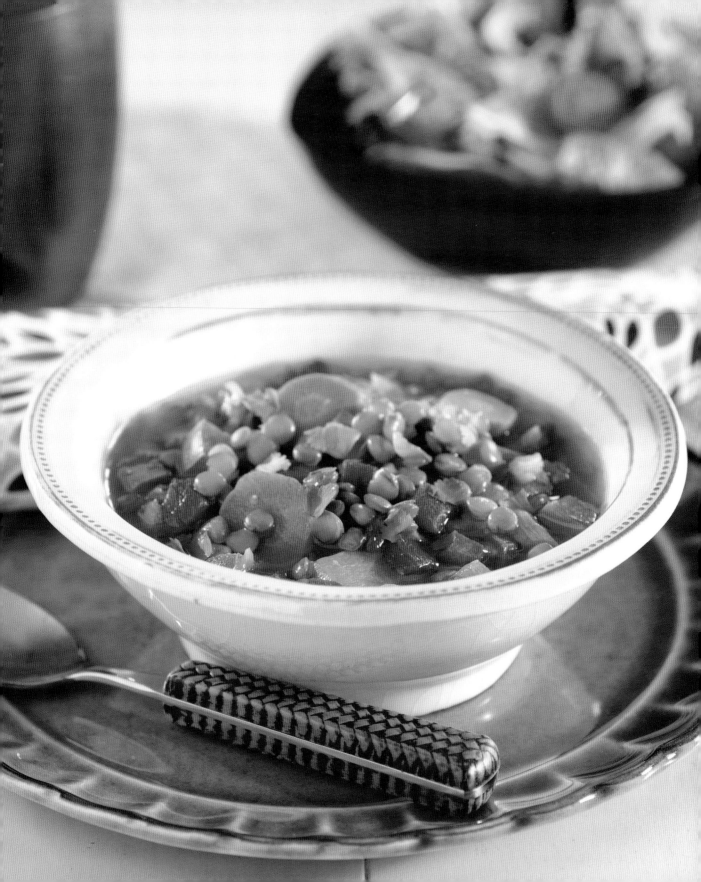

MIDDLE EASTERN SPINACH SALAD

¼ cup lemon juice

1 tablespoon olive oil

1 tablespoon packed light brown sugar

½ teaspoon curry powder

1 pound fresh spinach, torn into bite-size pieces

½ cup golden raisins

¼ cup minced red onion

¼ cup thin red onion slices

1. Whisk lemon juice, oil, brown sugar and curry powder in small bowl until blended; set aside.

2. Combine spinach, raisins, minced onion and onion slices in large bowl. Add dressing; gently toss to coat.

Makes 4 servings

Nutrients per Serving: ¾ *of total recipe*
Calories: 142, **Calories from Fat:** 22%, **Total Fat:** 4g, **Saturated Fat:** 1g, **Cholesterol:** 0mg, **Sodium:** 94mg, **Carbohydrate:** 27g, **Fiber:** 4g, **Protein:** 4g

TIP   To make ahead, prepare salad and dressing and store separately in refrigerator. Toss immediately before serving.

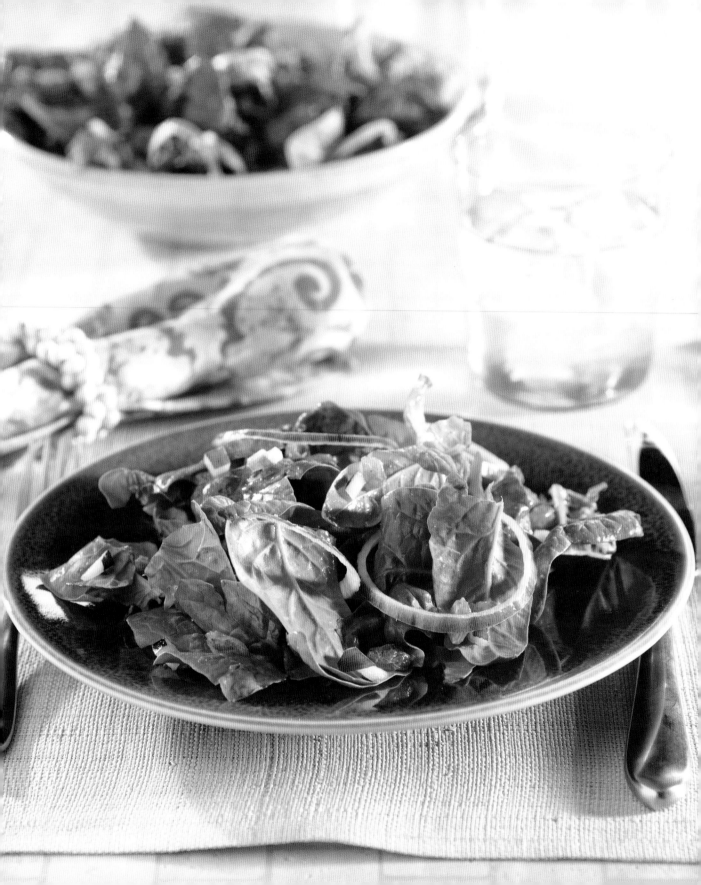

PUMPKIN SOUP WITH CRUMBLED BACON AND TOASTED PUMPKIN SEEDS

2 teaspoons olive oil

½ cup raw pumpkin seeds

1 onion, chopped

1 teaspoon kosher salt

½ teaspoon chipotle chili powder

½ teaspoon black pepper

2 cans (29 ounces each) solid-pack pumpkin

4 cups chicken stock or broth

¾ cup apple cider

½ cup whipping cream

Sour cream (optional)

3 slices thick-sliced bacon, crisp-cooked and crumbled

Slow Cooker Directions

1. Heat oil in medium nonstick skillet over medium heat. Add pumpkin seeds; cook and stir 1 minute or until seeds begin to pop. Remove to small bowl; cool completely.

2. Spray inside of slow cooker with nonstick cooking spray. Add onion to same skillet; cook and stir over medium heat until translucent. Stir in salt, chipotle powder and black pepper. Transfer to prepared slow cooker. Whisk in pumpkin, chicken stock and apple cider until smooth. Cover; cook on HIGH 4 hours.

3. Turn off slow cooker. Whisk in whipping cream. Strain soup through fine-mesh strainer; discard solids. Ladle soup into bowls; top evenly with sour cream, if desired, pumpkin seeds and bacon.

Makes 4 servings

Nutrients per Serving: *¼ of total recipe*
Calories: 220, **Calories from Fat:** 40%, **Total Fat:** 10g,
Saturated Fat: 2g, **Cholesterol:** 4mg, **Sodium:** 600mg,
Carbohydrate: 29g, **Fiber:** 13g, **Protein:** 10g

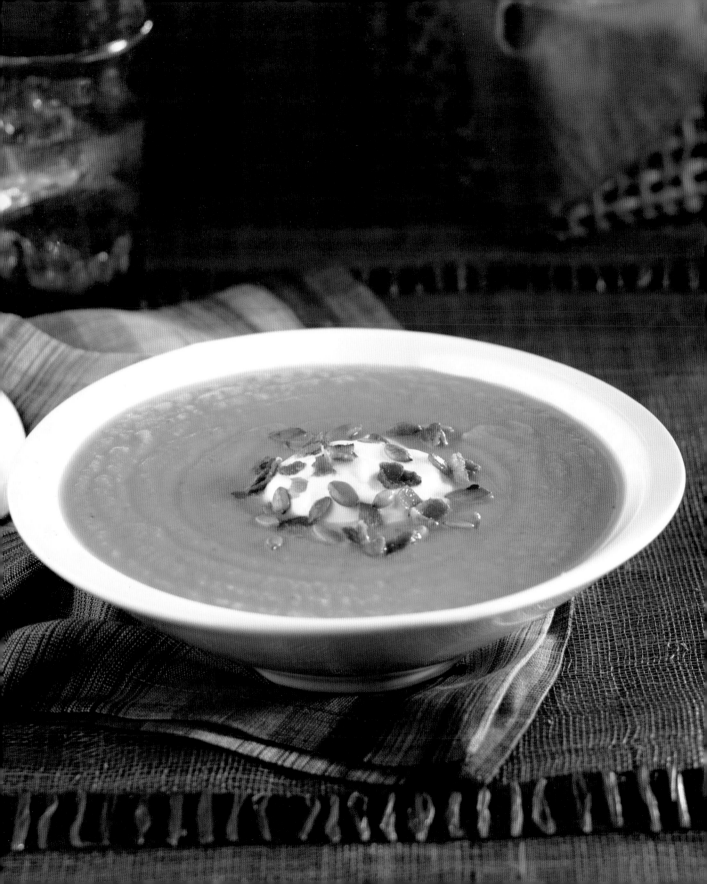

SPICY GRAPEFRUIT SALAD WITH RASPBERRY DRESSING

1 cup fresh or frozen thawed raspberries

2 tablespoons chopped green onion

1 teaspoon balsamic vinegar

1 tablespoon honey

½ teaspoon dry mustard

2 cups washed watercress

2 cups washed mixed salad greens

3 medium grapefruit, peeled, sectioned, seeded

½ pound jicama, cut into julienne strips

1. Reserve 12 raspberries for garnish. Combine remaining raspberries, green onion, vinegar, honey and mustard in food processor or blender; process until smooth. Set aside.

2. Combine watercress and salad greens; divide evenly among four plates. Arrange grapefruit and jicama evenly on top of greens. Drizzle evenly with dressing. Garnish with reserved raspberries.

Makes 4 servings

Nutrients per Serving: *¼ of total recipe*
Calories: 113, **Calories from Fat:** 5%, **Total Fat:** 1g,
Saturated Fat: 0g, **Cholesterol:** 0mg, **Sodium:** 16mg,
Carbohydrate: 26g, **Fiber:** 5g, **Protein:** 3g

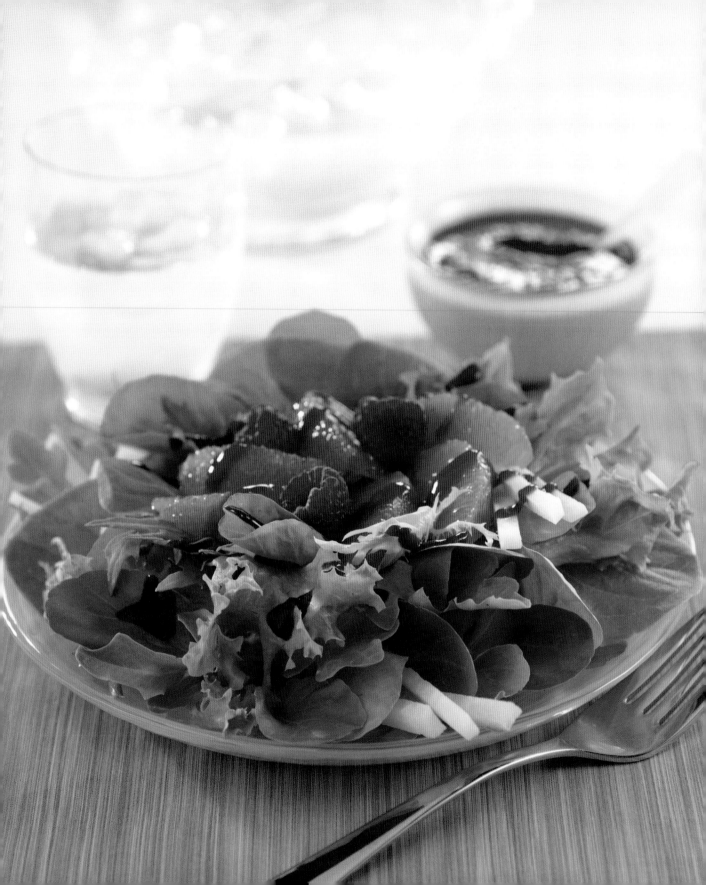

MEXICAN TORTILLA SOUP

Nonstick cooking spray

2 pounds boneless skinless chicken breasts, cut into ½-inch strips

4 cups diced carrots

2 cups sliced celery

1 cup chopped green bell pepper

1 cup chopped onion

4 cloves garlic, minced

1 jalapeño pepper,* sliced

1 teaspoon dried oregano

½ teaspoon ground cumin

8 cups fat-free reduced-sodium chicken broth

1 large tomato, chopped

4 to 5 tablespoons lime juice

2 (6-inch) corn tortillas, cut into ¼-inch strips

Salt (optional)

3 tablespoons finely chopped fresh cilantro

*Jalapeño peppers can sting and irritate the skin, so wear rubber gloves when handling peppers and do not touch your eyes.

1. Spray Dutch oven or large saucepan with cooking spray; heat over medium heat. Add chicken; cook and stir 10 minutes or until browned and cooked through.

2. Add carrots, celery, bell pepper, onion, garlic, jalapeño, oregano and cumin; cook and stir over medium heat 5 minutes. Add broth, tomato and lime juice; bring to a boil. Reduce heat to low; cover and simmer 15 to 20 minutes.

3. Meanwhile, preheat oven to 350°F. Arrange tortilla strips on baking sheet; spray lightly with cooking spray. Sprinkle lightly with salt, if desired. Bake 10 minutes or until browned and crisp, stirring occasionally.

continued on page 78

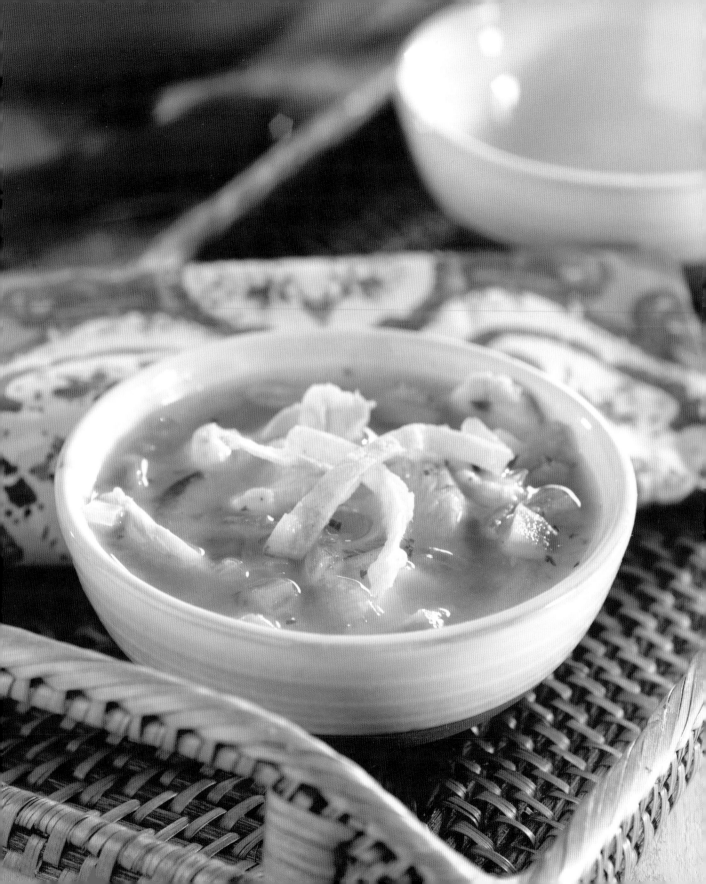

Mexican Tortilla Soup, continued

4. Stir cilantro into soup. Ladle soup into bowls; top evenly with tortilla strips.

Makes 8 servings

Nutrients per Serving: *1¾ cups with about ⅛ of tortilla strips*
Calories: 184, **Calories from Fat:** 15%, **Total Fat:** 3g,
Saturated Fat: 1g, **Cholesterol:** 58mg, **Sodium:** 132mg,
Carbohydrate: 16g, **Fiber:** 4g, **Protein:** 23g

TOMATO AND SUGAR SNAP SALAD

    8 ounces fresh sugar snap peas or green beans, trimmed
    2 medium tomatoes, cut into ½-inch wedges
    ¼ cup thinly sliced red onion
    2 tablespoons chopped fresh basil or parsley
    ¼ cup light balsamic salad dressing
    ¼ teaspoon salt
    ½ cup (2 ounces) crumbled reduced-fat feta cheese

1. Steam snap peas in steamer basket over boiling water 3 minutes or until crisp-tender. Immediately drain in colander; rinse with cold water until cool. Drain.

2. Combine snap peas, tomatoes, onion, basil, salad dressing and salt in medium bowl; gently toss to coat. Sprinkle with cheese; gently toss to coat.

Makes 8 servings

Nutrients per Serving: *¾ cup*
Calories: 60, **Calories from Fat:** 7%, **Total Fat:** 3g,
Saturated Fat: 1g, **Cholesterol:** 3mg, **Sodium:** 243mg,
Carbohydrate: 7g, **Fiber:** 2g, **Protein:** 5g

TOMATO AND SUGAR SNAP SALAD

CHICKEN BARLEY SOUP

1 teaspoon olive oil

1 package (8 ounces) sliced mushrooms

¾ cup chopped onion

¾ cup chopped carrot

¾ cup chopped celery

2 cloves garlic, minced

1 cup chopped cooked chicken

½ cup uncooked quick-cooking barley

1 bay leaf

¼ teaspoon dried thyme

¼ teaspoon black pepper

4 cups fat-free reduced-sodium chicken broth

Juice of 1 lemon

Parsley (optional)

1. Heat oil in Dutch oven or large saucepan over medium-high heat. Add mushrooms, onion, carrot, celery and garlic; cook and stir 5 minutes. Add chicken, barley, bay leaf, thyme and pepper. Pour in broth; bring to a boil. Reduce heat to low; cover and simmer 25 minutes or until vegetables are tender.

2. Remove and discard bay leaf; stir in lemon juice. Ladle soup into bowls; garnish with parsley.

Makes 8 servings

Nutrients per Serving: *1 cup*

Calories: 102, **Calories from Fat:** 9%, **Total Fat:** 1g, **Saturated Fat:** <1g, **Cholesterol:** 13mg, **Sodium:** 307mg, **Carbohydrate:** 15g, **Fiber:** 2g, **Protein:** 9g

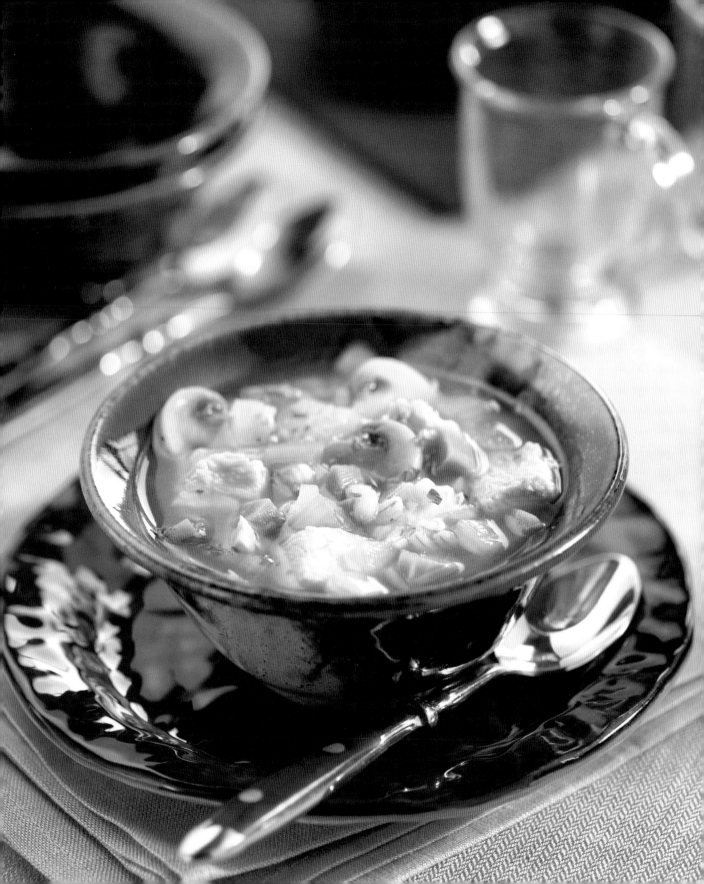

GREEK-STYLE CUCUMBER SALAD

1 medium cucumber, peeled and diced
¼ cup chopped green onions
1 teaspoon minced fresh dill
1 clove garlic, minced
1 cup sour cream or sour half-and-half
½ teaspoon salt
¼ teaspoon black pepper
⅛ teaspoon ground cumin
   Fresh lemon juice (optional)

1. Combine cucumber, green onions, dill and garlic in serving bowl.

2. Stir sour cream, salt, pepper and cumin in small bowl until well blended. Stir sour cream mixture into cucumber mixture. Sprinkle with lemon juice, if desired.

Makes 4 servings

Nutrients per Serving: *½ cup*
Calories: 116, **Calories from Fat:** 76%, **Total Fat:** 10g,
Saturated Fat: 6g, **Cholesterol:** 21mg, **Sodium:** 319mg,
Carbohydrate: 5g, **Fiber:** <1g, **Protein:** 2g

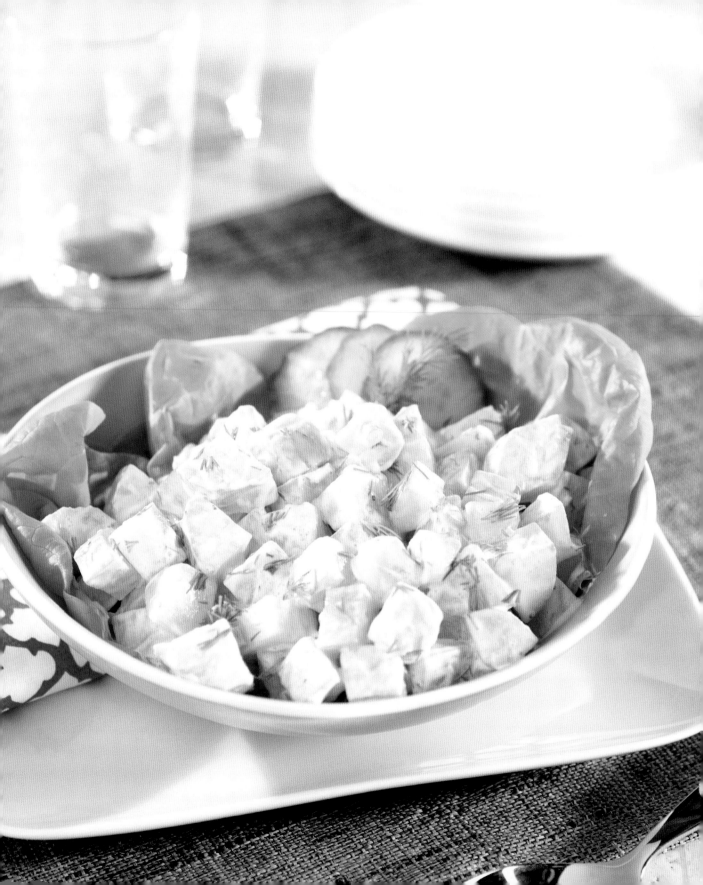

ITALIAN SKILLET ROASTED VEGETABLE SOUP

2 tablespoons olive oil, divided
1 medium red, yellow or orange bell pepper, chopped
1 clove garlic, minced
2 cups water
1 can (about 14 ounces) diced tomatoes
1 medium zucchini, thinly sliced lengthwise
⅛ teaspoon red pepper flakes
1 can (about 15 ounces) navy beans, rinsed and drained
3 to 4 tablespoons chopped fresh basil
1 tablespoon balsamic vinegar
½ teaspoon liquid smoke (optional)
¾ teaspoon salt

1. Heat 1 tablespoon oil in Dutch oven or large saucepan over medium-high heat. Add bell pepper; cook and stir 4 minutes or until edges are browned. Add garlic; cook and stir 15 seconds. Add water, tomatoes, zucchini and red pepper flakes. Bring to a boil over high heat. Reduce heat to low; cover and simmer 20 minutes.

2. Add beans, basil, remaining 1 tablespoon oil, vinegar, liquid smoke, if desired, and salt; simmer 5 minutes. Remove from heat; cover and let stand 10 minutes before serving.

Makes 5 servings

Nutrients per Serving: *1 cup*
Calories: 157, **Calories from Fat:** 18%, **Total Fat:** 3g,
Saturated Fat: <1g, **Cholesterol:** 0mg, **Sodium:** 670mg,
Carbohydrate: 25g, **Fiber:** 6g, **Protein:** 8g

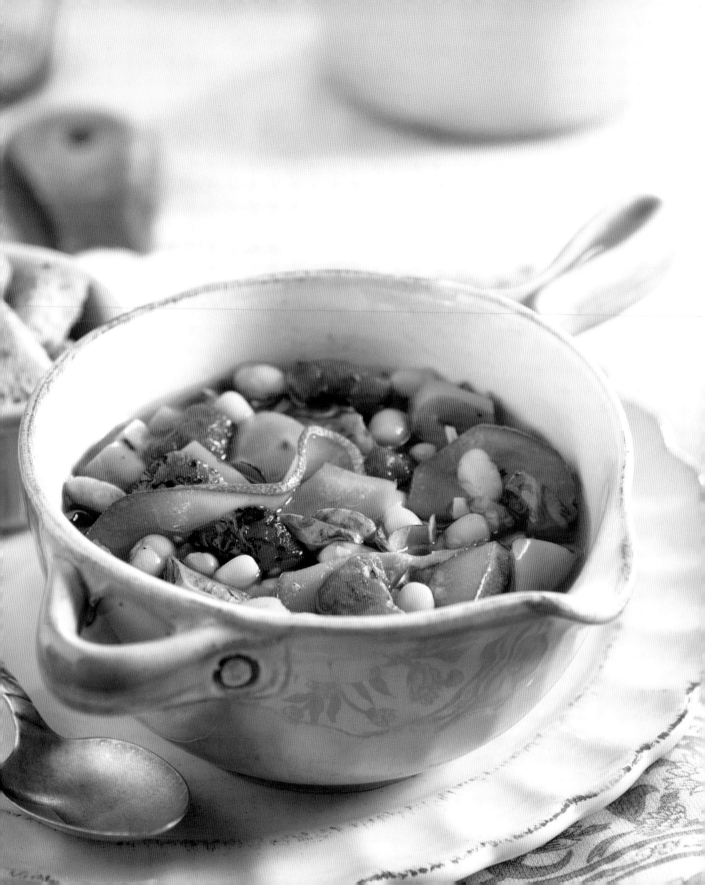

BLUEBERRY-ALMOND WALDORF SALAD

¼ cup plain low-fat yogurt

1 teaspoon honey

½ teaspoon whole grain or regular Dijon mustard

2 cups baby spinach

1 large Gala apple, cut into ½-inch pieces

1 large Granny Smith or Golden Delicious apple, cut into ½-inch pieces

½ cup fresh blueberries

¼ cup sliced almonds, toasted*

To toast almonds, spread in single layer in heavy-bottomed skillet. Cook over medium heat 1 to 2 minutes, stirring frequently, until lightly browned. Remove from skillet immediately. Cool before using.

Stir yogurt, honey and mustard in large bowl until smooth and well blended. Add spinach, apples, blueberries, and almonds; toss to coat. Serve immediately.

Makes 4 servings

Nutrients per Serving: *1 cup*
Calories: 107, **Calories from Fat:** 25%, **Total Fat:** 3g,
Saturated Fat: <1g, **Cholesterol:** 1mg, **Sodium:** 34mg,
Carbohydrate: 19g, **Fiber:** 4g, **Protein:** 3g

Note: This recipe is loaded with nutritional value. Almonds are best appreciated for their vitamin E content, heart-healthy monounsaturated fats and ability to stabilize blood sugar levels. Blueberries are packed with antioxidants and fiber. Spinach is also filled with antioxidants that act as anti-cancer agents.

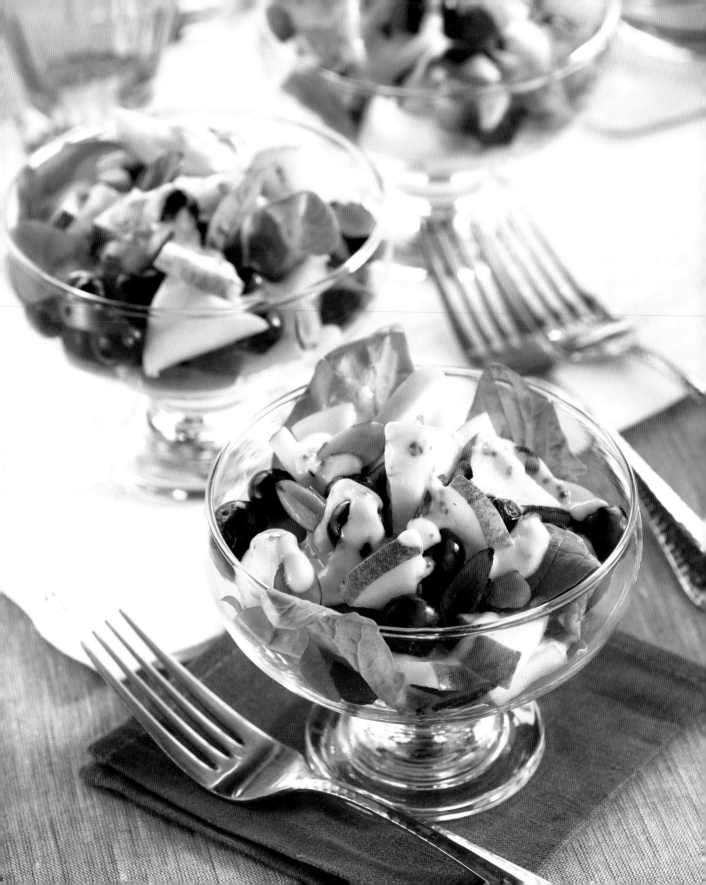

LUNCHES & LIGHT MEALS

CHICKEN, HUMMUS AND VEGETABLE WRAPS

- ¾ cup hummus (regular, roasted red pepper or roasted garlic)
- 4 (8- to 10-inch) sun-dried tomato, spinach or whole wheat tortillas
- 2 cups chopped cooked chicken breast
  Chipotle or Louisiana-style hot pepper sauce (optional)
- ½ cup shredded carrots
- ½ cup chopped unpeeled cucumber
- ½ cup thinly sliced radishes
- 2 tablespoons chopped fresh mint or basil

Spread hummus evenly over one side of tortillas. Arrange chicken over hummus; sprinkle with hot sauce, if desired. Top with carrots, cucumber, radishes and mint. Roll up to enclose filling; cut in half diagonally. *Makes 4 servings*

Nutrients per Serving: *1 wrap*
Calories: 308, **Calories from Fat:** 29%, **Total Fat:** 10g,
Saturated Fat: 1g, **Cholesterol:** 60mg, **Sodium:** 540mg,
Carbohydrate: 32g, **Fiber:** 15g, **Protein:** 32g

Variation: Substitute alfalfa sprouts for the radishes.

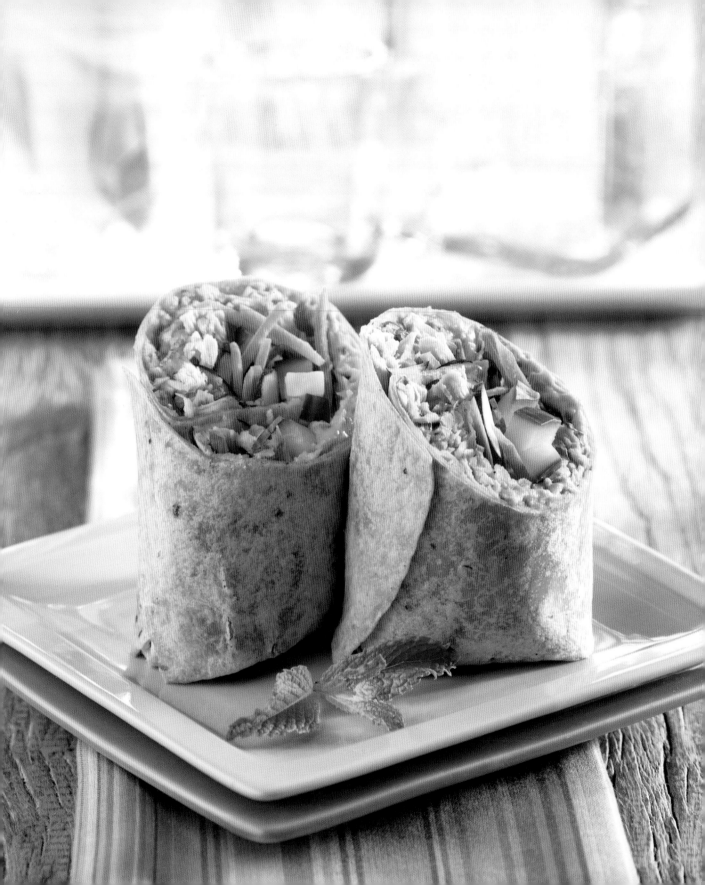

BEEF BURGERS WITH CORN SALSA

½ cup frozen corn

½ cup chopped tomato

1 can (about 4 ounces) diced green chiles, divided

1 tablespoon chopped fresh cilantro *or* 1 teaspoon dried cilantro

1 tablespoon white vinegar

1 teaspoon olive oil

¼ cup fine dry bread crumbs

3 tablespoons fat-free (skim) milk

¼ teaspoon garlic powder

12 ounces 95% lean ground beef

    Lettuce leaves

1. Prepare corn according to package directions; drain. Combine corn, tomato, 2 tablespoons chiles, cilantro, vinegar and oil in small bowl; toss to coat. Cover and refrigerate until ready to serve.

2. Preheat broiler. Combine bread crumbs, remaining chiles, milk and garlic powder in medium bowl; mix well. Add beef; mix lightly. Shape into four patties. Place on broiler pan.

3. Broil patties 4 inches from heat source 6 to 8 minutes. Turn over; broil 6 to 8 minutes or until cooked through (160°F). Serve on lettuce leaves with corn salsa.

Makes 4 servings

Nutrients per Serving: *1 burger with about*
1 tablespoon plus 2 teaspoons salsa
Calories: 180, **Calories from Fat:** 30%, **Total Fat:** 6g,
Saturated Fat: 2g, **Cholesterol:** 33mg, **Sodium:** 101mg,
Carbohydrate: 13g, **Fiber:** 2g, **Protein:** 19g

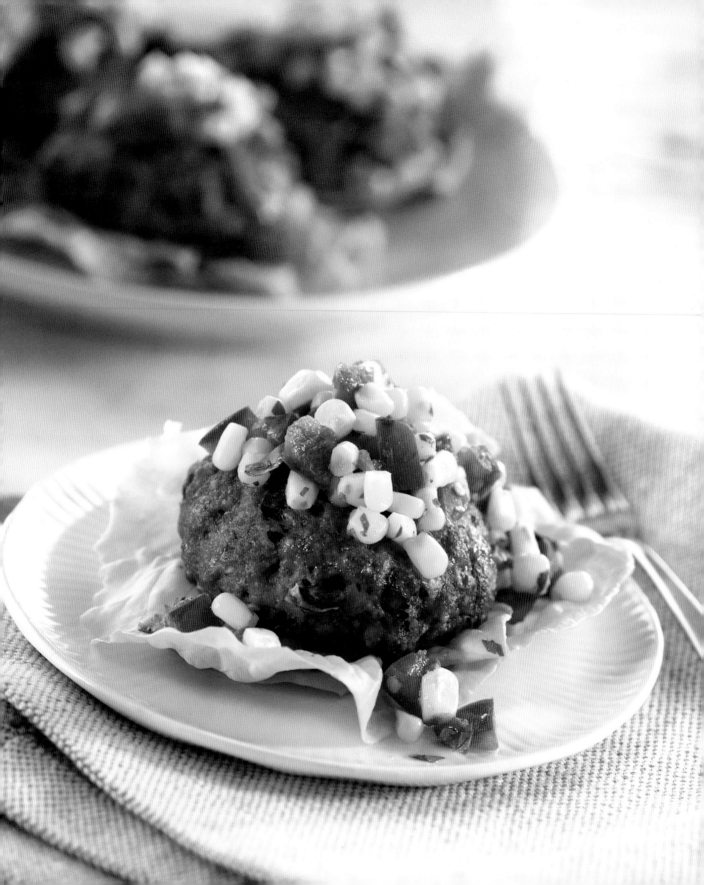

BROILED TUNA AND RASPBERRY SALAD

½ cup fat-free ranch salad dressing

¼ cup raspberry vinegar

1½ teaspoons Cajun seasoning

1 thick-sliced tuna steak (about 6 to 8 ounces)

2 cups torn romaine lettuce leaves

1 cup torn mixed baby lettuce leaves

½ cup fresh raspberries

1. Whisk salad dressing, vinegar and Cajun seasoning in small bowl until well blended. Pour ¼ cup dressing mixture into resealable food storage bag; reserve remaining dressing mixture. Add tuna to bag. Seal bag; turn to coat evenly. Marinate in refrigerator 10 minutes, turning once.

2. Preheat broiler. Spray rack of broiler pan with nonstick cooking spray. Place tuna on rack; reserve marinade. Broil tuna 4 inches from heat source 5 minutes. Turn over and brush with marinade; discard remaining marinade. Broil 5 minutes or until tuna flakes in center when tested with fork. Let stand 5 minutes.

3. Combine lettuces in large bowl; divide evenly among two serving plates. Cut tuna into ¼-inch-thick slices; arrange on salad. Top evenly with raspberries. Drizzle evenly with reserved dressing.

Makes 2 servings

Nutrients per Serving: *½ of total recipe*
Calories: 215, **Calories from Fat:** 22%, **Total Fat:** 5g,
Saturated Fat: 1g, **Cholesterol:** 35mg, **Sodium:** 427mg,
Carbohydrate: 18g, **Fiber:** 5g, **Protein:** 24g

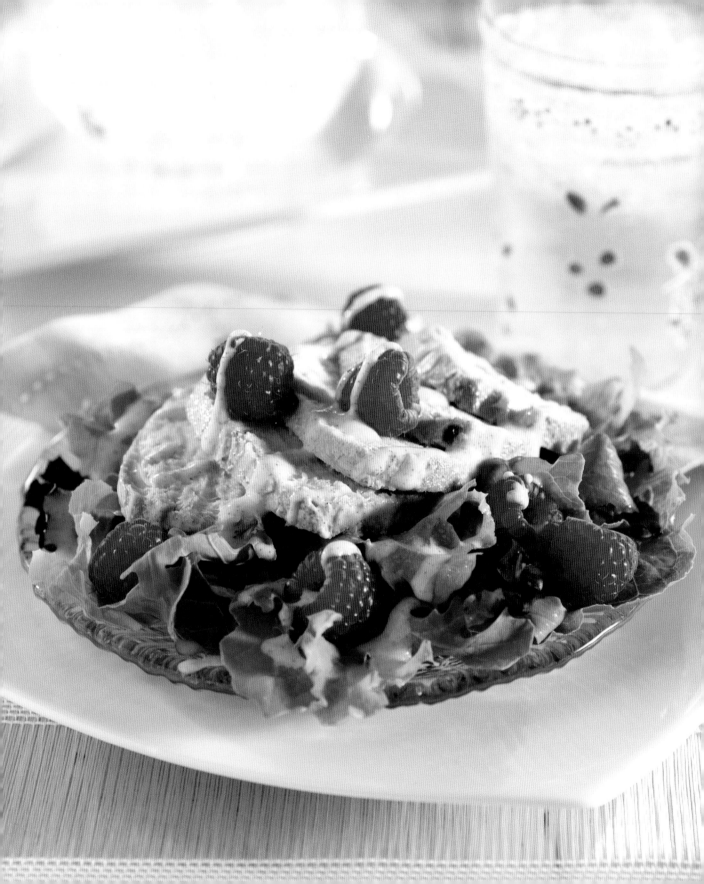

FALAFEL NUGGETS

Sauce

  2½ cups tomato sauce

  ⅓ cup tomato paste

  2 tablespoons lemon juice

  2 teaspoons sugar

  1 teaspoon onion powder

  ½ teaspoon salt

Falafel

  2 cans (about 15 ounces each) chickpeas

  ½ cup whole wheat flour

  ½ cup chopped fresh parsley

  1 egg, beaten

  Juice of 1 lemon

  ¼ cup minced onion

  2 tablespoons minced garlic

  2 teaspoons ground cumin

  ½ teaspoon salt

  ½ teaspoon ground red pepper or red pepper flakes

  ½ cup canola oil

1. Preheat oven to 400°F. Spray baking sheet with nonstick cooking spray.

2. Combine tomato sauce, tomato paste, 2 tablespoons lemon juice, sugar, onion powder and ½ teaspoon salt in medium saucepan. Simmer over medium-low heat 20 minutes or until heated through. Cover and keep warm until ready to serve.

3. Meanwhile, combine chickpeas, flour, parsley, egg, juice of 1 lemon, minced onion, garlic, cumin, ½ teaspoon salt and red pepper in food processor or blender; process until well blended. Shape mixture into 1-inch balls.

continued on page 96

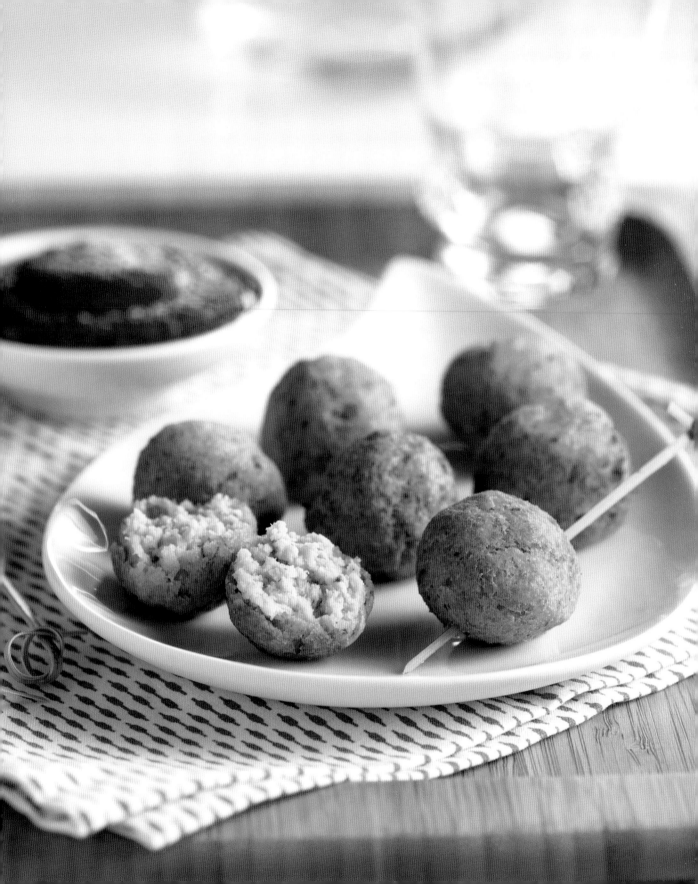

Falafel Nuggets, continued

4. Heat oil in large nonstick skillet over medium-high heat. Fry falafel in batches until browned. Using slotted spoon, remove from skillet and place 2 inches apart on prepared baking sheet.

5. Bake 8 to 10 minutes. Serve with warm sauce for dipping.   *Makes 12 servings*

Nutrients per Serving: *3 pieces falafel with about ¼ cup sauce*
Calories: 191, **Calories from Fat:** 34%, **Total Fat:** 7g,
Saturated Fat: 1g, **Cholesterol:** 0mg, **Sodium:** 701mg,
Carbohydrate: 26g, **Fiber:** 5g, **Protein:** 6g

Note: Falafel also can be baked completely to reduce fat content. Spray balls lightly with nonstick cooking spray and bake on baking sheet 15 to 20 minutes, turning once.

BLACK BEAN AND BELL PEPPER BURRITOS

  2 teaspoons canola oil
1½ cups diced assorted bell peppers
  ½ cup chopped onion
  1 can (about 15 ounces) black beans, rinsed and drained
  ½ cup salsa
  1 teaspoon chili powder
  7 (8-inch) whole wheat or multigrain low-carb flour tortillas, warmed
  ¾ cup (3 ounces) reduced-fat shredded Cheddar or Mexican cheese blend
  ½ cup chopped fresh cilantro

1. Heat oil in large nonstick skillet over medium heat. Add bell peppers and onion; cook and stir 3 to 4 minutes. Stir in beans, salsa and chili powder; cook and stir 5 to 8 minutes or until vegetables are tender.

2. Spoon about ⅔ cup bean mixture down center of each tortilla. Top evenly with cheese and cilantro. Roll up to enclose filling. *Makes 7 servings*

Nutrients per Serving: *1 burrito*
Calories: 170, **Calories from Fat:** 18%, **Total Fat:** 3.5g,
Saturated Fat: 1g, **Cholesterol:** 5mg, **Sodium:** 550mg,
Carbohydrate: 30g, **Fiber:** 6g, **Protein:** 10g

CURRIED LENTILS WITH FRUIT

   5 cups water
 1½ cups dried lentils, rinsed and sorted*
   1 Granny Smith apple, cored, peeled and chopped
   ¼ cup golden raisins
   ¼ cup lemon nonfat yogurt
   1 teaspoon curry powder
   1 teaspoon salt

*Packages of dried lentils may contain dirt and tiny stones. Thoroughly rinse lentils, then sort through them and discard any unusual looking pieces.

Slow Cooker Directions

1. Combine water, lentils, apple and raisins in slow cooker. Cover; cook on LOW 8 to 9 hours or until lentils are tender.**

2. Place lentil mixture in large serving bowl; stir in yogurt, curry powder and salt until well blended. *Makes 6 servings*

** Lentils should absorb most or all of the water. Slightly tilt slow cooker to check.

Nutrients per Serving: *½ cup*
Calories: 160, **Calories from Fat:** 3%, **Total Fat:** 1g,
Saturated Fat: <1g, **Cholesterol:** <1mg, **Sodium:** 364mg,
Carbohydrate: 31g, **Fiber:** 6g, **Protein:** 10g

GRILLED PIZZA WITH SPINACH AND ARTICHOKES

Nonstick cooking spray
2 cloves garlic, finely minced
3 cups fresh spinach leaves, coarsely chopped
1 (10-ounce) package prepared whole wheat thin pizza crust
½ cup prepared pizza sauce
1 cup chopped cooked chicken breast
½ cup chopped canned artichoke hearts, rinsed and drained
¾ cup shredded reduced-fat mozzarella cheese

1. Spray small nonstick skillet with cooking spray; heat over medium heat. Add garlic; cook and stir 30 seconds. Add spinach; cook and stir until spinach is wilted. Remove from heat; drain.

2. Place pizza crust on baking sheet. Spread sauce to within 1 inch of edge. Top evenly with spinach mixture, chicken, artichokes and cheese.

3. Prepare grill for indirect cooking. Transfer pizza to grill (do not put baking sheet on grill). Grill over medium heat 3 to 5 minutes or until cheese is melted and pizza is heated through. *Makes 6 servings*

Nutrients per Serving: *⅙ of total recipe*
Calories: 238, **Calories from Fat:** 26%, **Total Fat:** 7g,
Saturated Fat: 3g, **Cholesterol:** 24mg, **Sodium:** 460mg,
Carbohydrate: 28g, **Fiber:** 6g, **Protein:** 16g

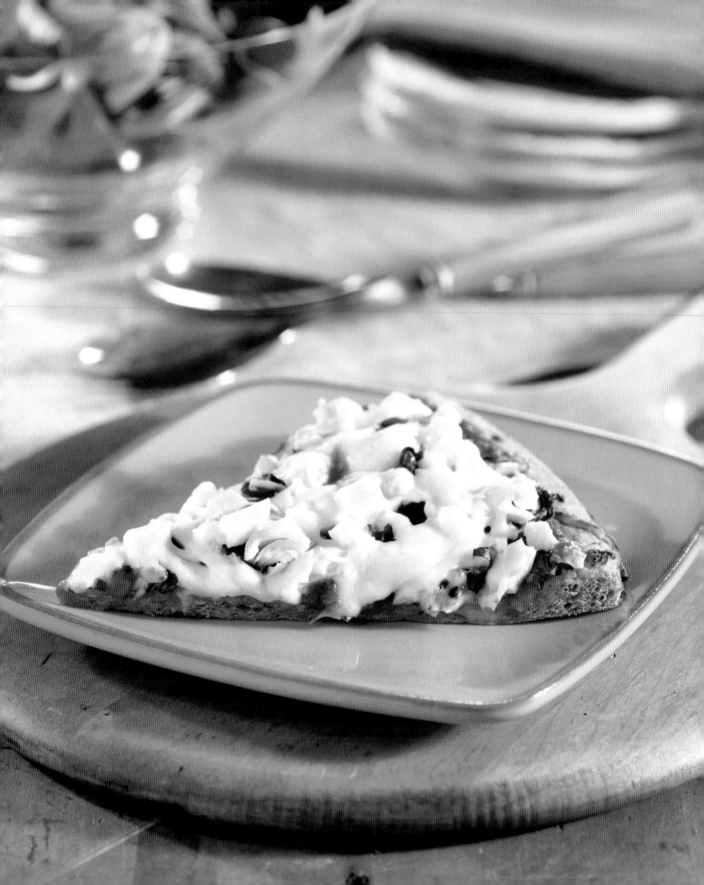

QUINOA AND SHRIMP SALAD

1 cup uncooked quinoa

2 cups water

½ teaspoon salt, divided

3 tablespoons olive oil

1 tablespoon lemon juice

1 teaspoon grated lemon peel

⅛ teaspoon black pepper

1 bag (12 ounces) cooked baby shrimp, thawed and well-drained

1 cup cherry or grape tomatoes, halved

¼ cup chopped fresh basil

2 tablespoons capers

2 tablespoons finely chopped green onion

1. Place quinoa in fine-mesh strainer; rinse well under cold running water. Bring water and ¼ teaspoon salt to a boil in medium saucepan; stir in quinoa. Cover; reduce heat to low. Simmer 12 to 14 minutes or until quinoa is tender and water is absorbed. Let stand 15 minutes, fluffing with fork occasionally.

2. Whisk oil, lemon juice, lemon peel, pepper and remaining ¼ teaspoon salt in small bowl until well blended. Combine quinoa, shrimp, tomatoes, basil, capers and green onion in large bowl. Pour dressing over quinoa mixture; gently toss to coat.

Makes 4 servings

Nutrients per Serving: *¼ of recipe*
Calories: 344, **Calories from Fat:** 36%, **Total Fat:** 14g,
Saturated Fat: 2g, **Cholesterol:** 166mg, **Sodium:** 620mg,
Carbohydrate: 32g, **Fiber:** 3g, **Protein:** 24g

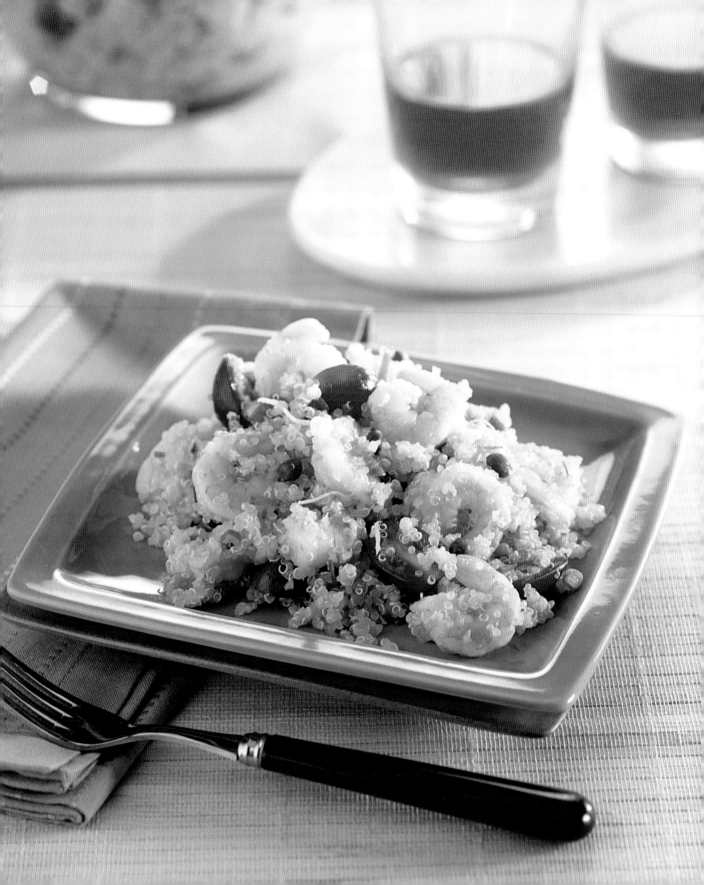

DELI BEEF WRAPS WITH CREAMY HONEY-MUSTARD SPREAD

3 tablespoons light mayonnaise

1 tablespoon honey mustard

1½ teaspoons packed dark brown sugar (optional)

4 whole grain or whole wheat tortillas

2 cups packed shredded lettuce

6 ounces thinly sliced deli roast beef

1 medium green bell pepper, thinly sliced

¼ cup thinly sliced red onion

1. Stir mayonnaise, honey mustard and brown sugar, if desired, in small bowl until well blended. Spread evenly on tortillas.

2. Layer lettuce, roast beef, bell pepper and onion evenly on tortillas. Roll up to enclose filling. Serve immediately or refrigerate up to 6 hours.   *Makes 4 wraps*

Nutrients per Serving: *1 wrap*
Calories: 245, **Calories from Fat:** 37%, **Total Fat:** 10g,
Saturated Fat: 2g, **Cholesterol:** 24mg, **Sodium:** 825mg,
Carbohydrate: 28g, **Fiber:** 2g, **Protein:** 11g

Variation: Stir chopped fresh cilantro into the mayonnaise mixture and add a layer of chopped avocado.

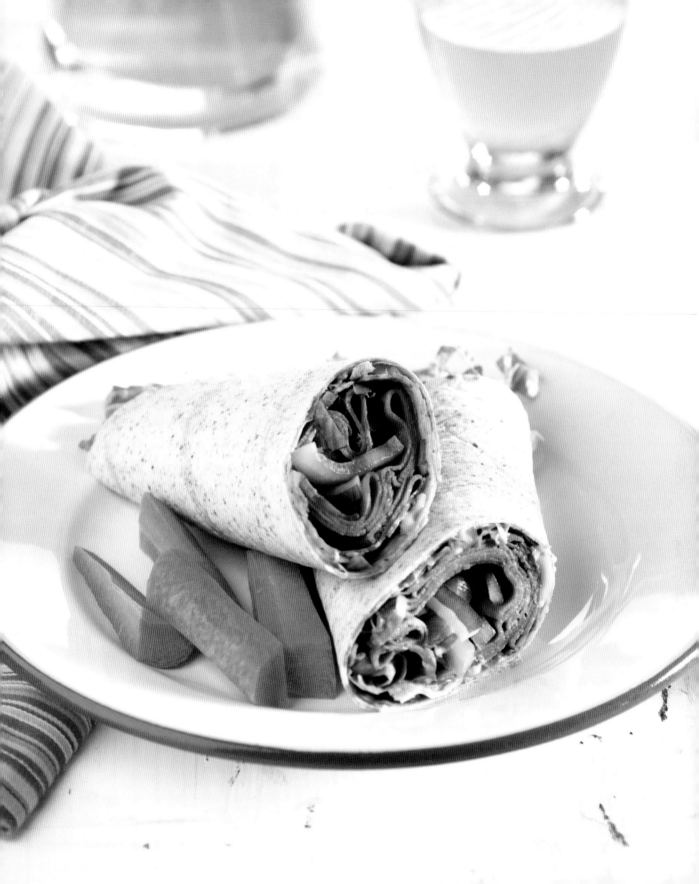

FRENCH LENTIL SALAD

2 quarts water

1½ cups dried lentils, rinsed and sorted*

4 green onions, finely chopped

3 tablespoons balsamic vinegar

2 tablespoons chopped fresh parsley

1 tablespoon olive oil

¾ teaspoon salt

½ teaspoon dried thyme

¼ teaspoon black pepper

Lettuce leaves (optional)

¼ cup chopped walnuts, toasted**

Packages of dried lentils may contain dirt and tiny stones. Thoroughly rinse lentils, then sort through them and discard any unusual looking pieces.

**To toast walnuts, spread in single layer in heavy-bottomed skillet. Cook over medium heat 1 to 2 minutes, stirring frequently until lightly browned. Remove from skillet immediately. Cool before using.*

1. Combine water and lentils in large saucepan; bring to a boil over high heat. Cover; reduce heat and simmer 30 minutes or until lentils are tender, stirring occasionally. Drain lentils; discard liquid.

2. Combine lentils, green onions, vinegar, parsley, oil, salt, thyme and pepper in large bowl; gently toss to combine. Cover and refrigerate 1 hour or until cool.

3. Serve salad on lettuce leaves, if desired. Top with walnuts just before serving.

Makes 4 servings

Nutrients per Serving: *¼ of total recipe*
Calories: 264, **Calories from Fat:** 28%, **Total Fat:** 8g,
Saturated Fat: 1g, **Cholesterol:** 0mg, **Sodium:** 406mg,
Carbohydrate: 34g, **Fiber:** 8g, **Protein:** 16g

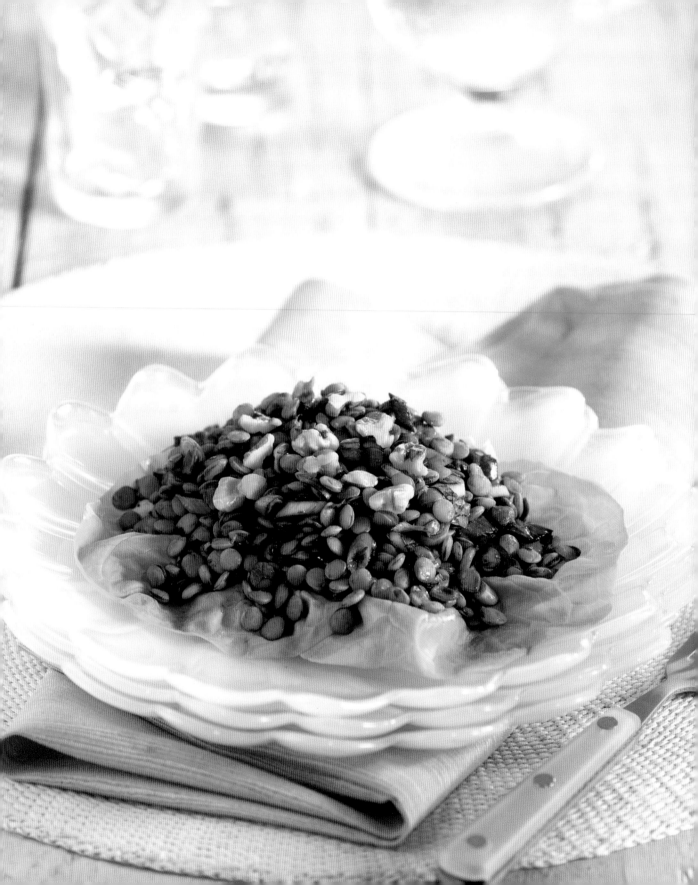

VEGGIE PIZZA PITAS

2 whole wheat pita bread rounds, cut in half horizontally
¼ cup prepared pizza sauce
1 teaspoon dried basil
⅛ teaspoon red pepper flakes (optional)
1 cup sliced mushrooms
½ cup thinly sliced green bell pepper
½ cup thinly sliced red onion
1 cup (4 ounces) shredded mozzarella cheese
2 teaspoons grated Parmesan cheese

1. Preheat oven to 475°F.

2. Arrange pita bread rounds, rough sides up, in single layer on baking sheet. Spread 1 tablespoon pizza sauce evenly over each round to within ¼ inch of edge. Sprinkle evenly with basil and red pepper flakes, if desired. Top evenly with mushrooms, bell pepper and onion. Sprinkle evenly with mozzarella cheese.

3. Bake 5 minutes or until cheese is melted. Sprinkle evenly with Parmesan cheese.

Makes 4 servings

Nutrients per Serving: *1 pizza*
Calories: 113, **Calories from Fat:** 18%, **Total Fat:** 2g,
Saturated Fat: 1g, **Cholesterol:** 6mg, **Sodium:** 402mg,
Carbohydrate: 13g, **Fiber:** 2g, **Protein:** 11g

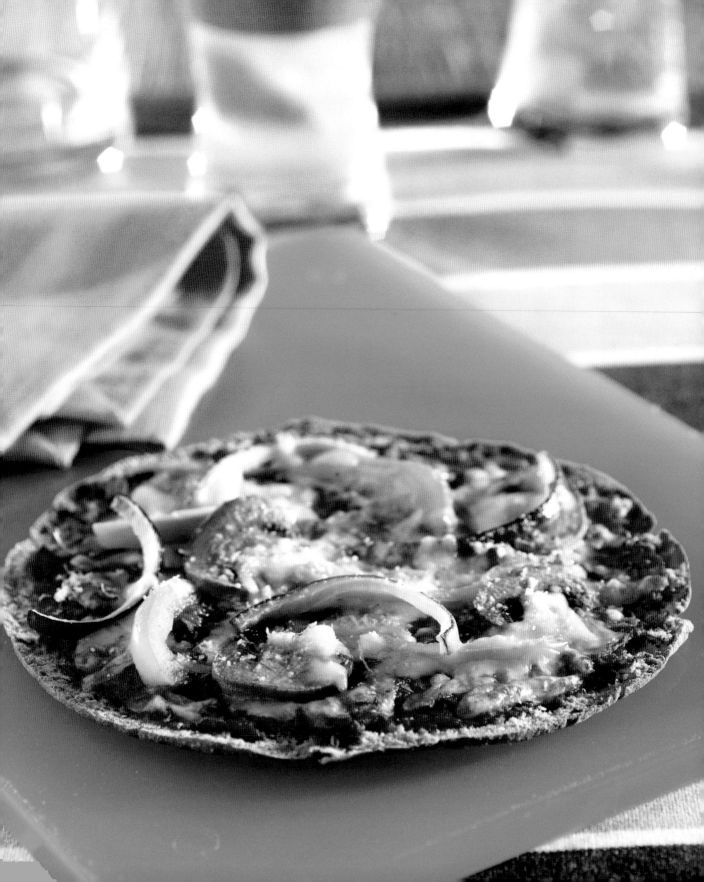

ZESTY TACO SALAD

2 tablespoons canola oil

1 tablespoon red wine vinegar

1 clove garlic, minced

¾ pound 93% lean ground turkey

1¾ teaspoons chili powder

¼ teaspoon ground cumin

3 cups torn lettuce leaves

1 can (about 14 ounces) Mexican-style diced tomatoes, drained

1 cup canned chickpeas or pinto beans, rinsed and drained

⅔ cup chopped peeled cucumber

⅓ cup frozen corn, thawed

¼ cup chopped red onion

1 jalapeño pepper,* finely chopped (optional)

12 fat-free tortilla chips

Mixed greens (optional)

*Jalapeño peppers can sting and irritate the skin, so wear rubber gloves when handling peppers and do not touch your eyes.

1. Whisk oil, vinegar and garlic in small bowl until well blended; set aside.

2. Combine turkey, chili powder and cumin in large nonstick skillet. Cook over medium heat 5 minutes or until turkey is cooked through and no longer pink, stirring to break up meat.

3. Combine turkey, lettuce, tomatoes, chickpeas, cucumber, corn, onion and jalapeño, if desired, in large bowl. Add dressing; toss to coat. Serve on greens, if desired, with tortilla chips.

Makes 4 servings

Nutrients per Serving: *1½ cups salad with 3 tortilla chips*
Calories: 285, **Calories from Fat:** 33%, **Total Fat:** 11g,
Saturated Fat: 1g, **Cholesterol:** 33mg, **Sodium:** 484mg,
Carbohydrate: 28g, **Fiber:** 5g, **Protein:** 21g

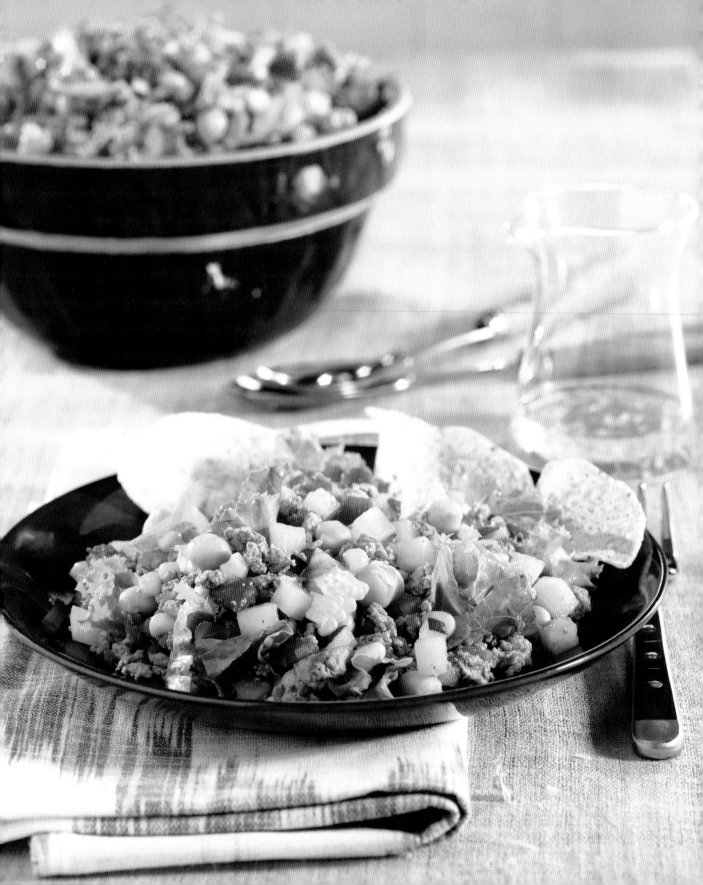

OPEN-FACED REUBENS

1 cup shredded cabbage

2 tablespoons reduced-fat mayonnaise, divided

2 tablespoons reduced-sodium or no-salt-added chili sauce, divided

4 slices pumpernickel or rye bread, toasted

4 ounces sliced pastrami

2 slices reduced-fat Swiss cheese, cut into ½-inch strips

1. Preheat broiler. Combine cabbage, 1 tablespoon mayonnaise and 1 tablespoon chili sauce in medium bowl; toss to coat.

2. Stir remaining 1 tablespoon mayonnaise and 1 tablespoon chili sauce in small bowl until well blended. Spread mayonnaise mixture over half of bread slices. Top each with 1 ounce pastrami, ¼ cup cabbage mixture and one fourth of cheese strips. Place on baking sheet.

3. Broil 4 to 5 inches from heat source 40 seconds to 1 minute or until cheese is melted.

Makes 4 servings

Nutrients per Serving: *1 sandwich*
Calories: 164, **Calories from Fat:** 22%, **Total Fat:** 4g,
Saturated Fat: 2g, **Cholesterol:** 24mg, **Sodium:** 670mg,
Carbohydrate: 21g, **Fiber:** 3g, **Protein:** 12g

Note: Cabbage is in the same family as kale, Brussels sprouts, broccoli and collard greens. It's an excellent source of vitamin C and a very good source of fiber, folic acid and omega-3 fatty acids.

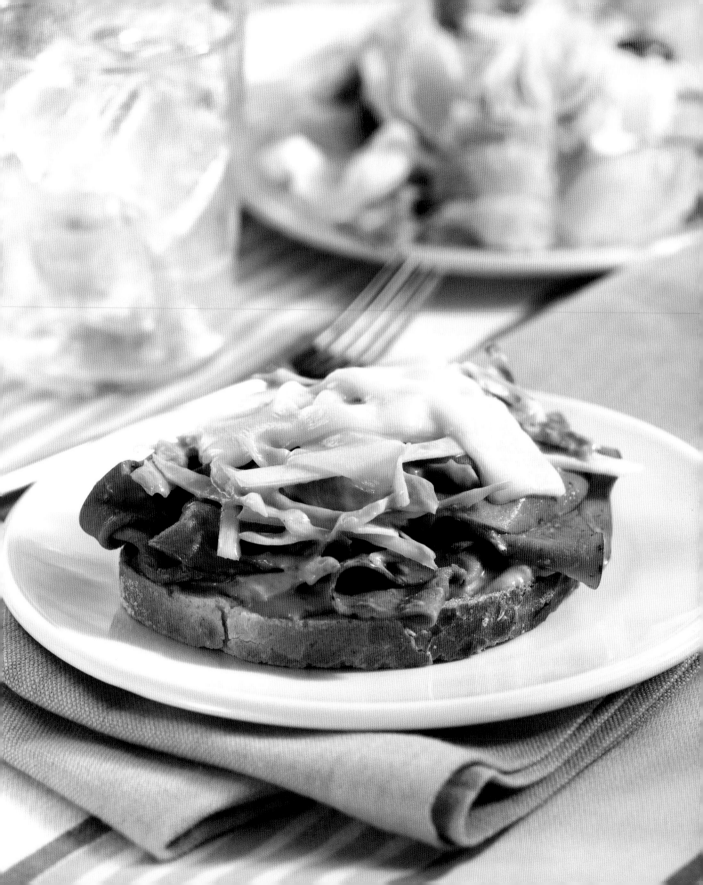

FAJITA PILE-UPS

2 teaspoons vegetable oil, divided
¾ pound beef top sirloin steak, trimmed of fat, cut into thin strips
2 teaspoons salt-free steak seasoning
½ medium lime
1 medium green bell pepper, cut into ½-inch strips
1 medium red or yellow bell pepper, cut into ½-inch strips
1 large onion, cut into ½-inch wedges
1 cup cherry tomatoes, halved
½ teaspoon ground cumin
4 (6-inch) corn tortillas, warmed
½ cup fat-free sour cream
2 tablespoons chopped fresh cilantro (optional)
    Lime wedges (optional)

1. Heat 1 teaspoon oil in large nonstick skillet over medium-high heat. Add steak; sprinkle with seasoning. Cook and stir 3 minutes or just until slightly pink in center. *Do not overcook.* Transfer to plate. Squeeze lime juice over steak. Cover to keep warm.

2. Add remaining 1 teaspoon oil to skillet. Add bell peppers and onion; cook and stir 8 minutes or until tender. Add tomatoes; cook and stir 1 minute. Return steak and any accumulated juices and cumin to skillet; cook and stir 1 minute.

3. Arrange tortillas on serving plates; top evenly with steak mixture and sour cream. Garnish with cilantro and lime wedges.   *Makes 4 servings*

Nutrients per Serving: *1¼ cups steak mixture with 1 tortilla*
Calories: 252, **Calories from Fat:** 24%, **Total Fat:** 7g,
Saturated Fat: 2g, **Cholesterol:** 41mg, **Sodium:** 90mg,
Carbohydrate: 24g, **Fiber:** 4g, **Protein:** 24g

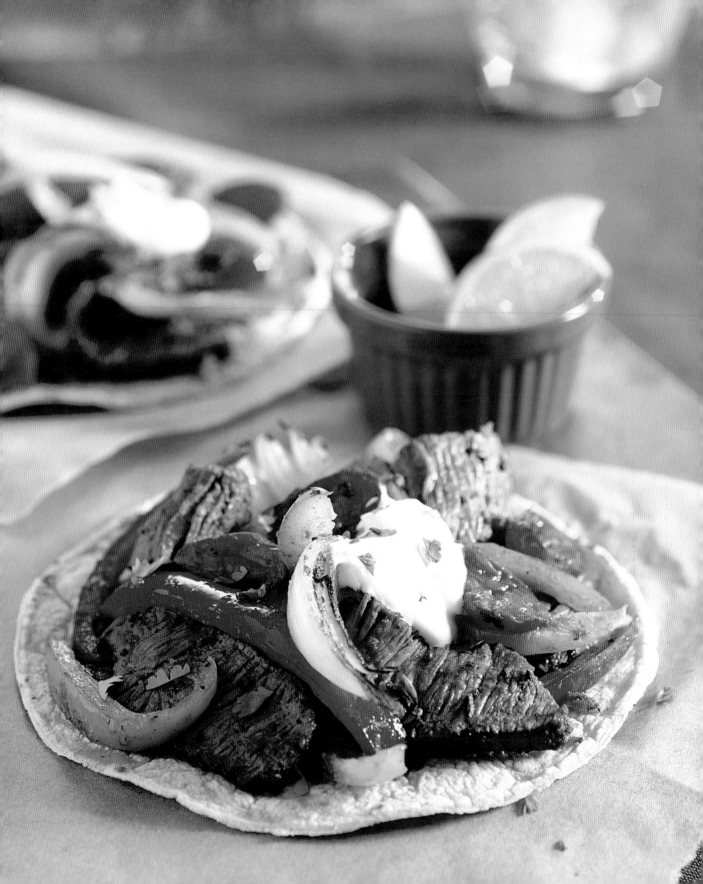

MEDITERRANEAN SANDWICHES

       Nonstick cooking spray
1¼ pounds chicken tenders, cut crosswise in half
  1 large tomato, cut into bite-size pieces
 ½ small cucumber, halved lengthwise, seeded and sliced
 ½ cup sweet onion slices (about 1 small)
  2 tablespoons cider vinegar
  1 tablespoon olive or canola oil
  3 teaspoons minced fresh oregano *or* ½ teaspoon dried oregano
  2 teaspoons minced fresh mint *or* ¼ teaspoon dried mint
 ¼ teaspoon salt
 12 lettuce leaves (optional)
  6 (6-inch) whole wheat pita bread rounds, cut in half crosswise

1. Spray large nonstick skillet with cooking spray; heat over medium heat. Add chicken; cook and stir 7 to 10 minutes or until browned and cooked through. Let stand to cool slightly.

2. Combine chicken, tomato, cucumber and onion in medium bowl. Drizzle with vinegar and oil; toss to coat. Sprinkle with oregano, mint and salt; toss to combine.

3. Place 1 lettuce leaf in each pita bread half, if desired. Divide chicken mixture evenly among pita bread halves.   *Makes 6 servings*

Nutrients per Serving: *2 filled pita halves*
Calories: 242, **Calories from Fat:** 21%, **Total Fat:** 6g,
Saturated Fat: 1g, **Cholesterol:** 50mg, **Sodium:** 353mg,
Carbohydrate: 24g, **Fiber:** 2g, **Protein:** 23g

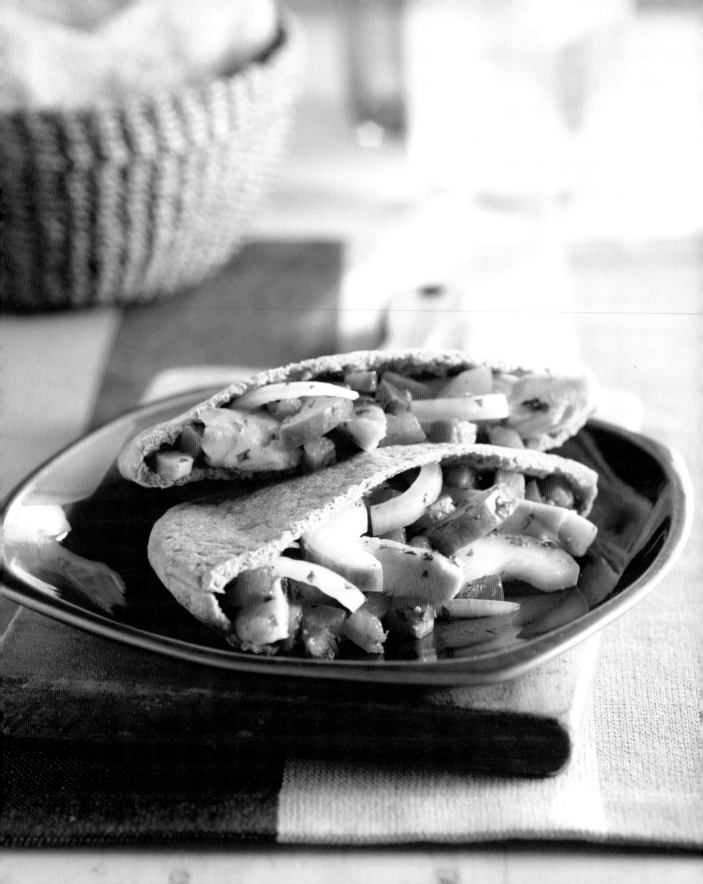

BULGUR SALAD NIÇOISE

 2 cups water
¼ teaspoon salt
 1 cup uncooked bulgur
1½ tablespoons lemon juice, or to taste
 1 tablespoon olive oil
⅛ teaspoon black pepper
 1 cup halved cherry tomatoes
 1 can (6 ounces) tuna packed in water, drained and flaked
½ cup pitted black niçoise olives*
 3 tablespoons finely chopped green onions, green part only
 1 tablespoon chopped fresh mint leaves (optional)
   Mint leaves (optional)

*If using larger olives, slice or chop as desired.

1. Bring water and salt to a boil in medium saucepan. Stir in bulgur. Remove from heat. Cover and let stand 10 to 15 minutes or until bulgur is tender and water is absorbed. Fluff with fork; set aside to cool completely.

2. Whisk lemon juice, oil and pepper in small bowl until well blended. Combine bulgur, tomatoes, tuna, olives, green onions and chopped mint, if desired, in large bowl. Pour dressing over bulgur mixture; gently toss to combine. Garnish with mint leaves, if desired.

Makes 3 servings

Nutrients per Serving: *⅓ of total recipe*
Calories: 307, **Calories from Fat:** 23%, **Total Fat:** 8g,
Saturated Fat: 1g, **Cholesterol:** 17mg, **Sodium:** 593mg,
Carbohydrate: 40g, **Fiber:** 10g, **Protein:** 21g

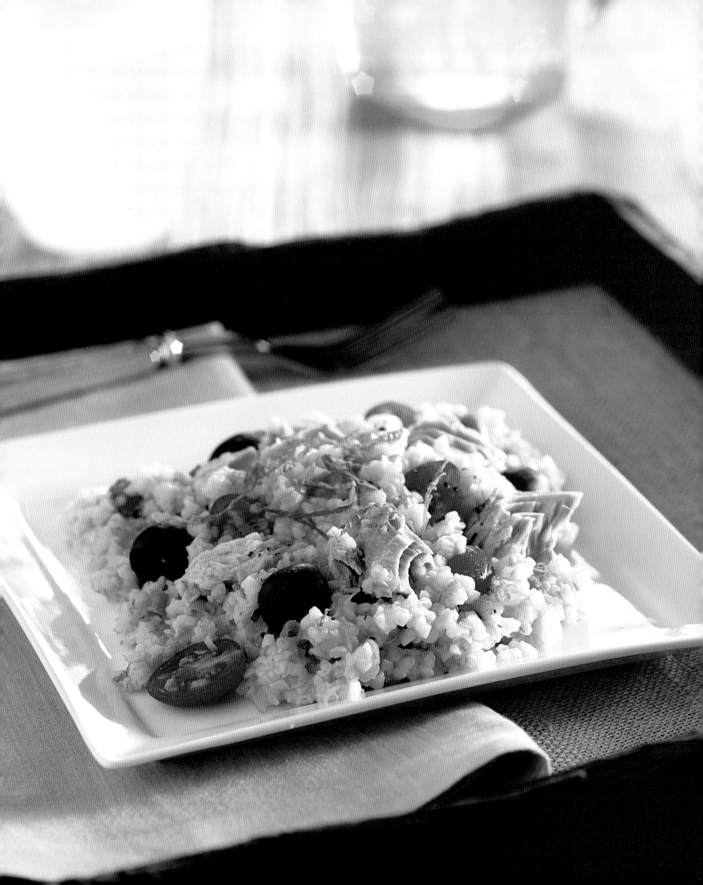

HOISIN BARBECUE CHICKEN SLIDERS

⅔ cup hoisin sauce

⅓ cup barbecue sauce

3 tablespoons quick-cooking tapioca

1 tablespoon sugar

1 tablespoon reduced-sodium soy sauce

¼ teaspoon red pepper flakes

12 boneless, skinless chicken thighs (3 to 3½ pounds total)

16 dinner rolls or Hawaiian sweet rolls, split

½ medium red onion, finely chopped

Sliced pickles (optional)

Slow Cooker Directions

1. Combine hoisin sauce, barbecue sauce, tapioca, sugar, soy sauce and red pepper flakes in slow cooker; mix well. Add chicken. Cover; cook on LOW 8 to 9 hours.

2. Remove chicken from sauce. Coarsely shred with two forks. Return shredded chicken and any sauce to slow cooker; mix well.

3. Spoon ¼ cup chicken and sauce on each bun. Serve with chopped red onion and pickles, if desired.

Makes 16 sliders

Nutrients per Serving: *1 slider*
Calories: 280, **Calories from Fat:** 29%, **Total Fat:** 8g,
Saturated Fat: 3g, **Cholesterol:** 75mg, **Sodium:** 500mg,
Carbohydrate: 35g, **Fiber:** 13g, **Protein:** 22g

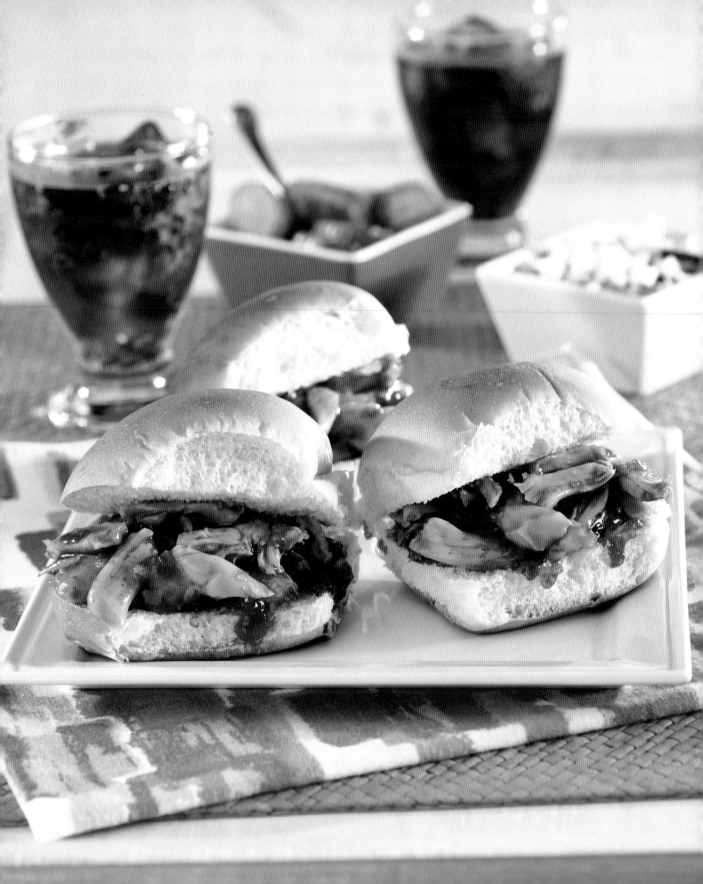

ZESTY VEGETARIAN CHILI

1 tablespoon canola or vegetable oil
1 large red bell pepper, finely chopped
2 medium zucchini or yellow squash (or 1 of each), cut into ½-inch chunks
4 cloves garlic, minced
1 can (about 14 ounces) fire-roasted diced tomatoes
¾ cup chunky salsa
2 teaspoons chili powder
1 teaspoon dried oregano
1 can (about 15 ounces) no-salt-added red kidney beans, rinsed and drained
10 ounces extra-firm tofu, well drained and cut into ½-inch cubes
   Chopped cilantro (optional)

1. Heat oil in large saucepan over medium heat. Add bell pepper; cook and stir 4 minutes. Add zucchini and garlic; cook and stir 3 minutes. Stir in tomatoes, salsa, chili powder and oregano; bring to a boil over high heat. Reduce heat to low; simmer 15 minutes or until vegetables are tender.

2. Stir beans into chili. Simmer 2 minutes or until heated through. Stir in tofu; remove from heat. Ladle chili into bowls; garnish with cilantro.   *Makes 4 servings*

Nutrients per Serving: *1½ cups*
Calories: 231, **Calories from Fat:** 31%, **Total Fat:** 8g,
Saturated Fat: 1g, **Cholesterol:** 0mg, **Sodium:** 432mg,
Carbohydrate: 28g, **Fiber:** 8g, **Protein:** 15g

Note: Tofu is made from the curds of soybean milk. It has a bland, slightly nutty taste, but readily takes on the flavor of foods it's cooked with. It's available in three forms: soft, firm and extra-firm. Cover any leftover tofu with water and refrigerate.

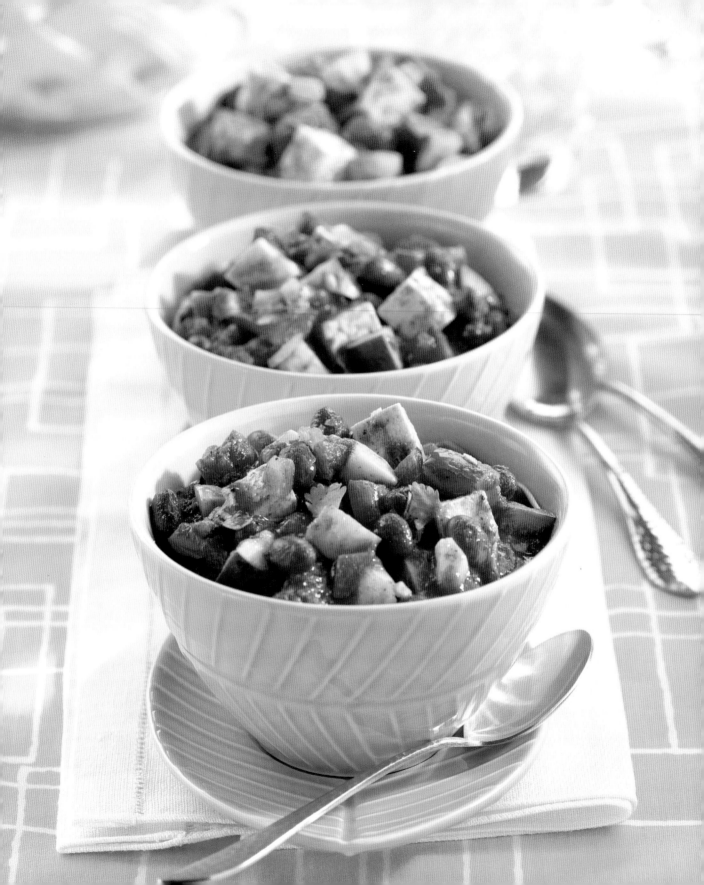

MAIN DISHES

STEAK DIANE WITH CREMINI MUSHROOMS

Nonstick cooking spray

2 beef tenderloin steaks, cut ¾ inch thick (about 4 ounces each)

¼ teaspoon black pepper

⅓ cup sliced shallots or chopped onion

4 ounces cremini mushrooms, sliced *or* 1 (4-ounce) package sliced mixed wild mushrooms

1½ tablespoons Worcestershire sauce

1 tablespoon Dijon mustard

1. Spray large nonstick skillet with cooking spray; heat over medium-high heat. Add steaks; sprinkle with pepper. Cook 3 minutes per side or until desired doneness. Transfer to plate; cover to keep warm.

2. Spray same skillet with cooking spray; heat over medium heat. Add shallots; cook and stir 2 minutes. Add mushrooms; cook and stir 3 minutes. Add Worcestershire sauce and mustard; cook and stir 1 minute.

3. Return steaks and any accumulated juices to skillet; cook until heated through, turning once. Serve steaks with mushroom mixture. *Makes 2 servings*

Nutrients per Serving: *½ of total recipe*
Calories: 239, **Calories from Fat:** 35%, **Total Fat:** 9g,
Saturated Fat: 3g, **Cholesterol:** 70mg, **Sodium:** 302mg,
Carbohydrate: 10g, **Fiber:** 1g, **Protein:** 28g

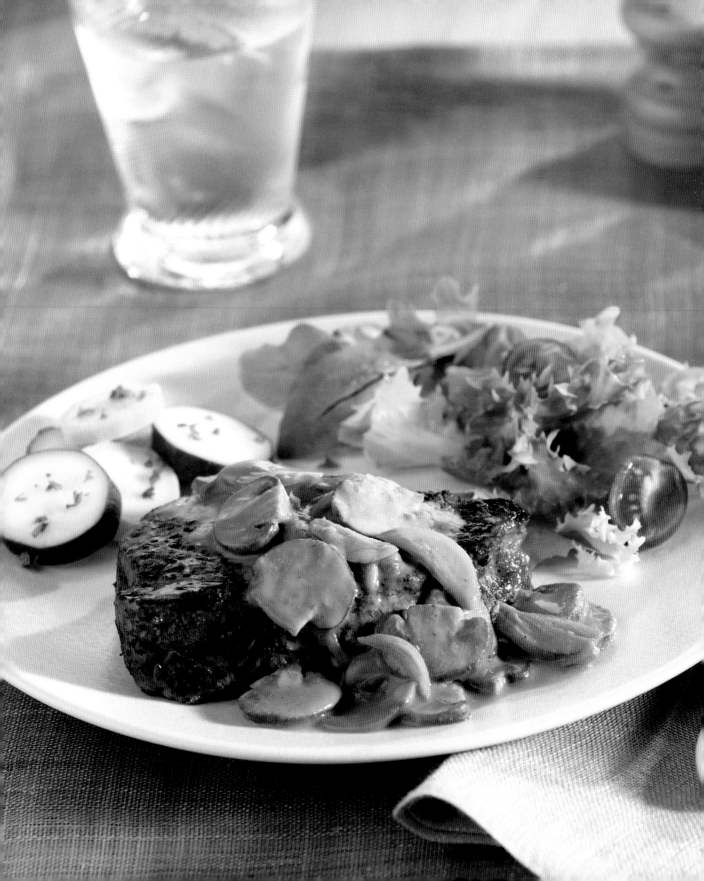

THAI-STYLE PORK KABOBS

⅓ cup reduced-sodium soy sauce
2 tablespoons fresh lime juice
2 tablespoons water
2 teaspoons hot chili oil*
2 cloves garlic, minced
1 teaspoon minced fresh ginger
12 ounces well-trimmed pork tenderloin, cut into ½-inch strips
1 red or yellow bell pepper, cut into ½-inch pieces
1 red or sweet onion, cut into ½-inch chunks
2 cups hot cooked rice

*Or combine 2 teaspoons vegetable oil and ½ teaspoon red pepper flakes in small microwavable bowl. Microwave on HIGH 30 to 45 seconds. Let stand 5 minutes to allow flavors to develop.

1. Whisk soy sauce, lime juice, water, chili oil, garlic and ginger in medium bowl until well blended. Reserve ⅓ cup for dipping sauce. Add pork to remaining soy sauce mixture; toss to coat evenly. Cover; refrigerate at least 30 minutes or up to 2 hours, turning once.

2. Meanwhile, soak eight 8- to 10-inch wooden skewers in cold water 30 minutes (to prevent burning).

3. Spray grid with nonstick cooking spray. Prepare grill for direct cooking. Remove pork; discard marinade. Thread pork, bell pepper and onion onto skewers.

4. Grill kabobs, covered, over medium heat 6 to 8 minutes or until pork is barely pink in center, turning halfway through grilling time. Serve with rice and reserved dipping sauce.   *Makes 4 servings*

Nutrients per Serving: *2 kabobs with ½ cup rice*
and about 1 tablespoon plus 1 teaspoon dipping sauce
Calories: 248, **Calories from Fat:** 16%, **Total Fat:** 4g,
Saturated Fat: 1g, **Cholesterol:** 49mg, **Sodium:** 271mg,
Carbohydrate: 30g, **Fiber:** 2g, **Protein:** 22g

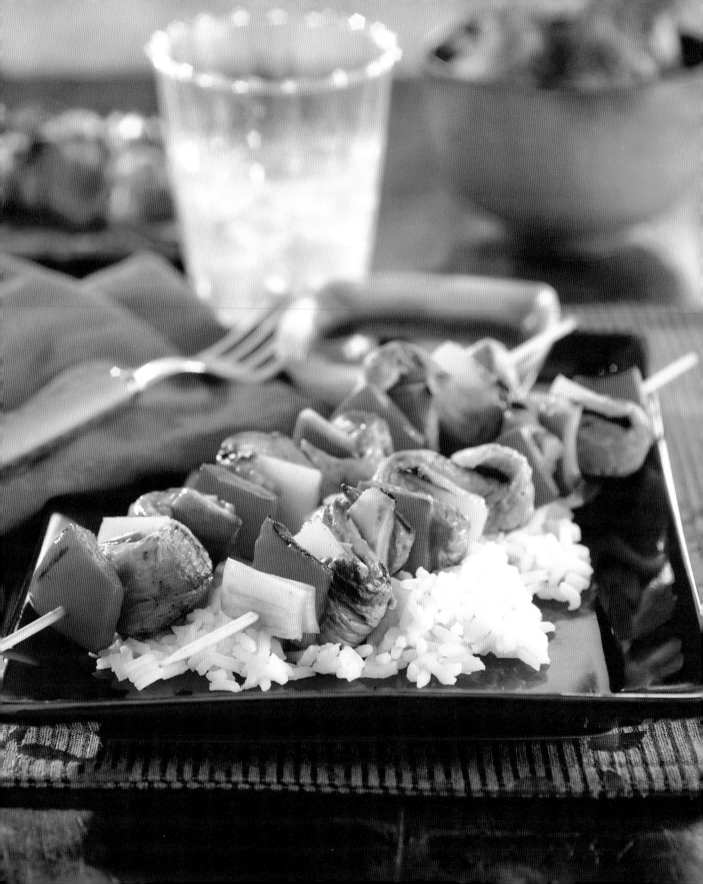

TURKEY BREAST WITH BARLEY-CRANBERRY STUFFING

2 cups reduced-sodium chicken broth

1 cup uncooked quick-cooking barley

½ cup chopped onion

½ cup dried cranberries

2 tablespoons slivered almonds, toasted*

½ teaspoon rubbed sage

½ teaspoon garlic-pepper seasoning

   Nonstick cooking spray

1 fresh or thawed frozen bone-in turkey breast half (about 2 pounds), skin removed

⅓ cup finely chopped fresh parsley

To toast almonds, spread in single layer in heavy-bottomed skillet. Cook over medium heat 1 to 2 minutes, stirring frequently, until lightly browned. Remove from skillet immediately. Cool before using.

Slow Cooker Directions

1. Combine broth, barley, onion, cranberries, almonds, sage and seasoning in slow cooker.

2. Spray large nonstick skillet with cooking spray; heat over medium heat. Brown turkey on all sides. Transfer to slow cooker. Cover; cook on LOW 4 to 6 hours.

3. Transfer turkey to cutting board; tent with foil and let stand 10 to 15 minutes before slicing.

4. Stir parsley into stuffing. Serve sliced turkey with stuffing. *Makes 6 servings*

Nutrients per Serving: ⅙ *of total recipe*
Calories: 298, **Calories from Fat:** 13%, **Total Fat:** 5g, **Saturated Fat:** 1g, **Cholesterol:** 55mg, **Sodium:** 114mg, **Carbohydrate:** 33g, **Fiber:** 6g, **Protein:** 31g

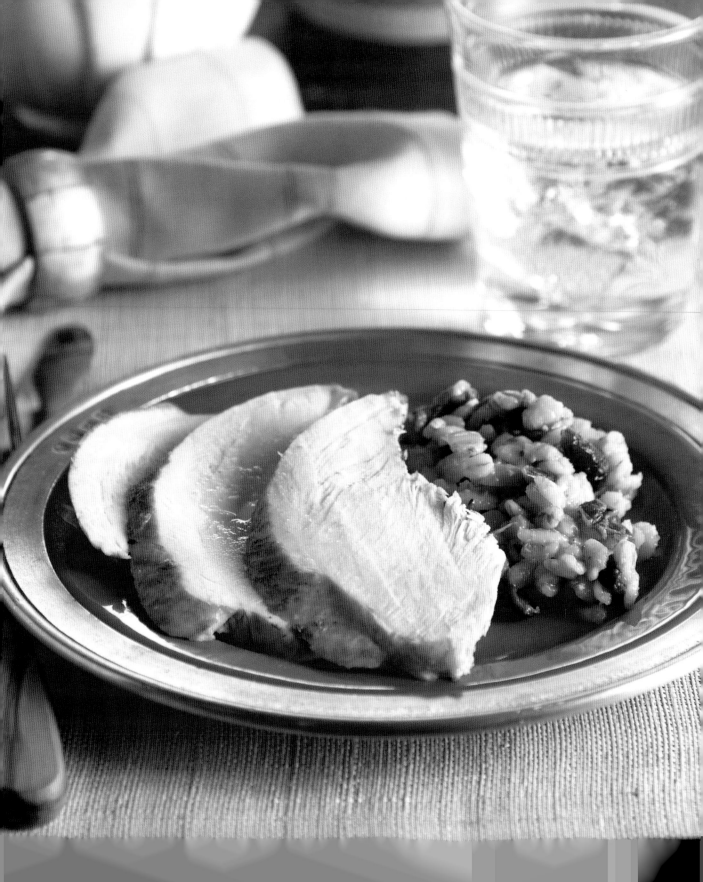

WHOLE WHEAT PENNE WITH BROCCOLI AND SAUSAGE

6 ounces uncooked whole wheat penne pasta

8 ounces broccoli florets (about 2 cups)

8 ounces mild Italian turkey sausage, casings removed

1 medium onion, quartered and sliced

2 cloves garlic, minced

2 teaspoons grated lemon peel

¼ teaspoon salt

⅛ teaspoon black pepper

⅓ cup grated Parmesan cheese

1. Cook pasta according to package directions. Add broccoli during last 5 to 6 minutes of cooking. Drain; cover and keep warm.

2. Meanwhile, heat large nonstick skillet over medium heat. Crumble sausage into skillet. Add onion; cook until sausage is brown, stirring to break up meat. Drain fat. Add garlic; cook and stir 1 minute.

3. Add sausage mixture, lemon peel, salt and pepper to pasta and broccoli; toss to combine. Divide evenly among six serving plates; sprinkle evenly with cheese.

Makes 6 servings

Nutrients per Serving: *1⅓ cups*
Calories: 208, **Calories from Fat:** 27%, **Total Fat:** 6g,
Saturated Fat: 1g, **Cholesterol:** 26mg, **Sodium:** 425mg,
Carbohydrate: 26g, **Fiber:** 4g, **Protein:** 13g

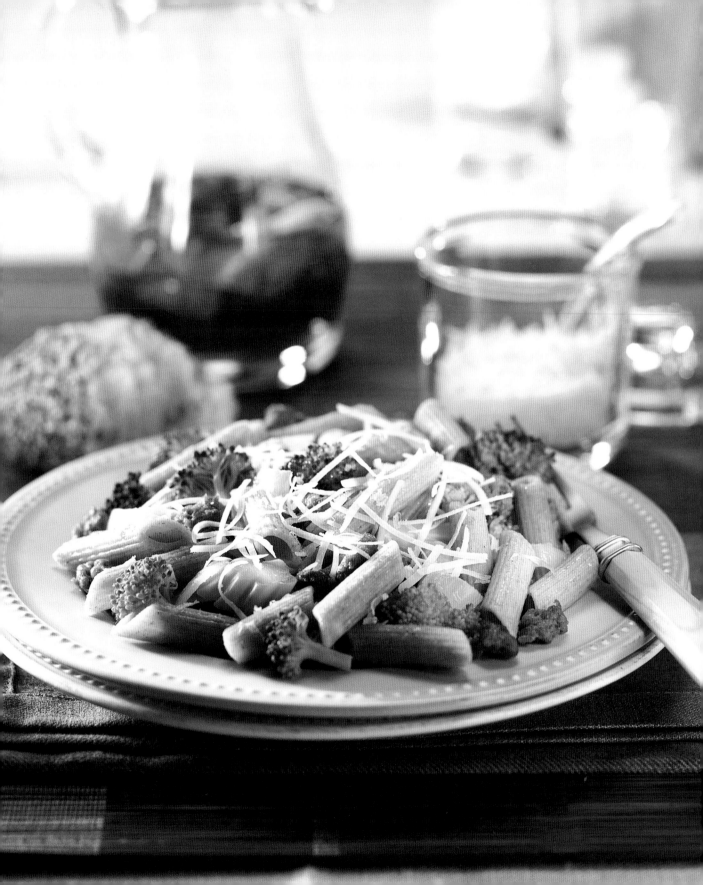

CHICKEN PICCATA

3 tablespoons all-purpose flour

½ teaspoon salt

¼ teaspoon black pepper

4 boneless skinless chicken breasts (4 ounces each)

2 teaspoons olive oil

1 teaspoon butter

2 cloves garlic, minced

¾ cup fat-free reduced-sodium chicken broth

1 tablespoon fresh lemon juice

2 tablespoons chopped fresh Italian parsley

1 tablespoon capers, drained

1. Combine flour, salt and pepper in shallow dish. Reserve 1 tablespoon flour mixture.

2. Pound chicken between waxed paper to ½-inch thickness with flat side of meat mallet or rolling pin. Coat chicken with remaining flour mixture, shaking off excess.

3. Heat oil and butter in large nonstick skillet over medium heat. Add chicken; cook 4 to 5 minutes per side or until no longer pink in center. Transfer to serving platter; tent loosely with foil.

4. Add garlic to same skillet; cook and stir 1 minute. Add reserved 1 tablespoon flour mixture; cook and stir 1 minute. Add broth and lemon juice; cook 2 minutes or until thickened, stirring frequently. Stir in parsley and capers.

5. Remove foil and spoon sauce over chicken. Serve immediately.   *Makes 4 servings*

Nutrients per Serving: *1 chicken breast with about ¼ cup sauce*
Calories: 194, **Calories from Fat:** 30%, **Total Fat:** 6g,
Saturated Fat: 2g, **Cholesterol:** 71mg, **Sodium:** 473mg,
Carbohydrate: 5g, **Fiber:** <1g, **Protein:** 27g

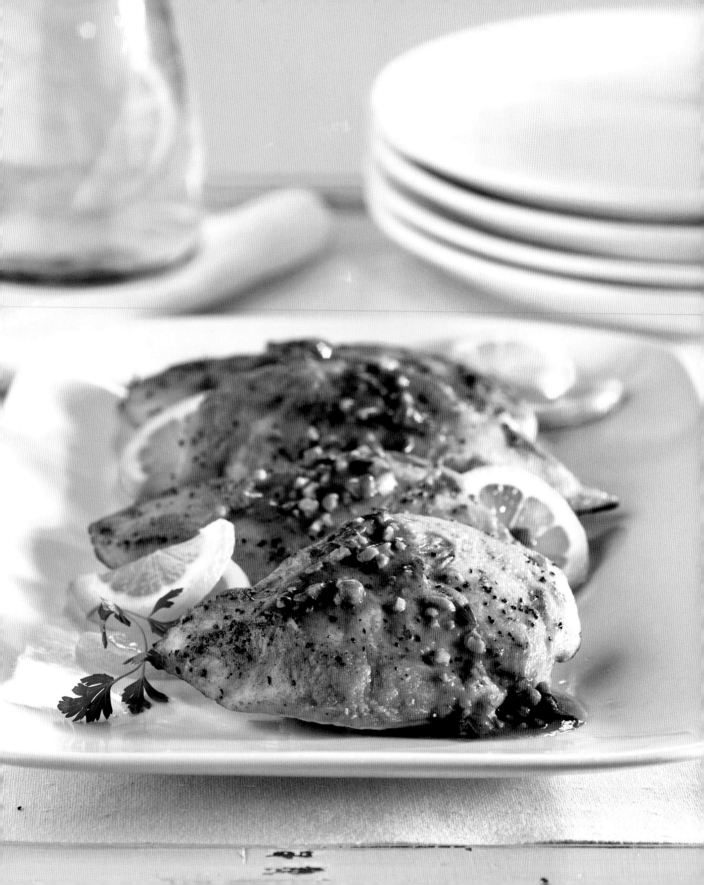

SWEET POTATO SHEPHERD'S PIE

1 large sweet potato, peeled and cubed

1 large russet potato, peeled and cubed

¼ cup fat-free (skim) milk

¾ teaspoon salt

1 pound 93% lean ground turkey

2 packages (4 ounces each) sliced mixed mushrooms *or*
    8 ounces sliced cremini mushrooms

1 jar (12 ounces) beef gravy

½ teaspoon dried thyme

¼ teaspoon black pepper

¾ cup frozen baby peas, thawed

    Nonstick cooking spray

1. Place potatoes in medium saucepan. Cover with water; bring to a boil over medium-high heat. Reduce heat; cover and simmer 20 minutes or until potatoes are very tender. Drain potatoes; return to saucepan. Mash with potato masher; stir in milk and salt until well blended.

2. Crumble turkey into large nonstick ovenproof skillet. Add mushrooms; cook and stir over medium-high heat until turkey is no longer pink and mushrooms begin to give off liquid. Drain.

3. Combine turkey mixture, gravy, thyme and pepper in same skillet; simmer 5 minutes. Add peas; cook and stir until heated through. Remove from heat. Spoon potato mixture over turkey mixture; spray with cooking spray.

4. Preheat broiler. Broil 4 to 5 inches from heat source 5 minutes or until mixture is heated through and potatoes begin to brown.   *Makes 6 servings*

Nutrients per Serving: *⅙ of total recipe*
Calories: 188, **Calories from Fat:** 12%, **Total Fat:** 3g,
Saturated Fat: 1g, **Cholesterol:** 32mg, **Sodium:** 689mg,
Carbohydrate: 19g, **Fiber:** 3g, **Protein:** 23g

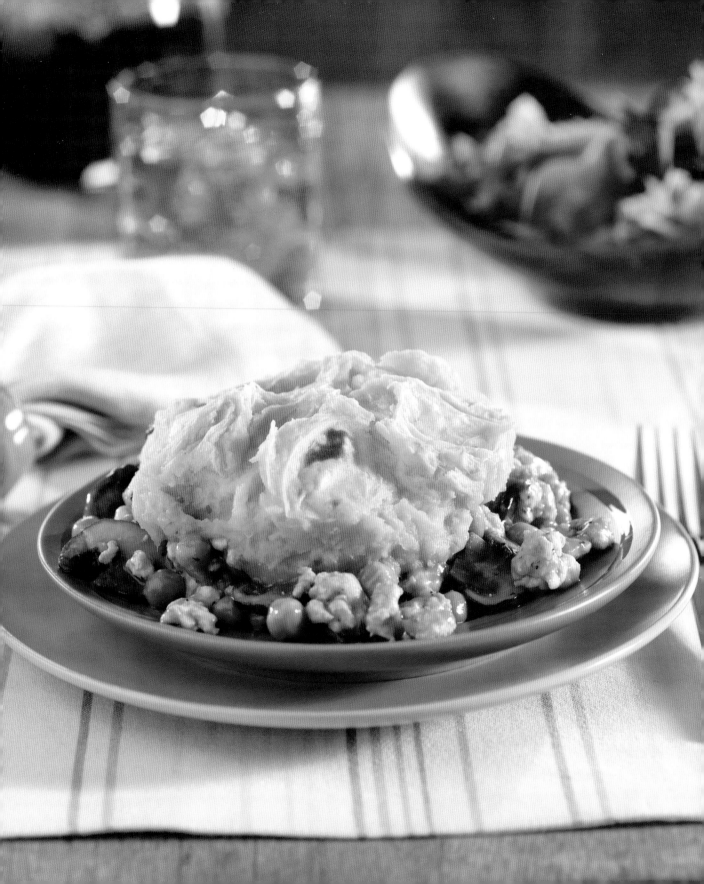

TUNA STEAKS WITH PINEAPPLE AND TOMATO SALSA

1 medium tomato, chopped

1 can (8 ounces) pineapple chunks in juice, drained and chopped

1 jalapeño pepper,* minced

2 tablespoons chopped fresh cilantro

1 tablespoon minced red onion

2 teaspoons lime juice

½ teaspoon grated lime peel

4 tuna steaks (4 ounces each)

½ teaspoon salt

⅛ teaspoon black pepper

2 teaspoons olive oil

Jalapeño peppers can sting and irritate the skin, so wear rubber gloves when handling peppers and do not touch your eyes.

1. Combine tomato, pineapple, jalapeño, cilantro, onion, lime juice and lime peel in medium bowl; gently toss. Set aside.

2. Sprinkle tuna with salt and pepper. Heat oil in large nonstick skillet over medium-high heat. Add tuna; cook 2 to 3 minutes per side or until desired doneness. Serve with salsa.

Makes 4 servings

Nutrients per Serving: *1 tuna steak with about ½ cup salsa*
Calories: 228, **Calories from Fat:** 32%, **Total Fat:** 8g,
Saturated Fat: 2g, **Cholesterol:** 43mg, **Sodium:** 338mg,
Carbohydrate: 11g, **Fiber:** 1g, **Protein:** 27g

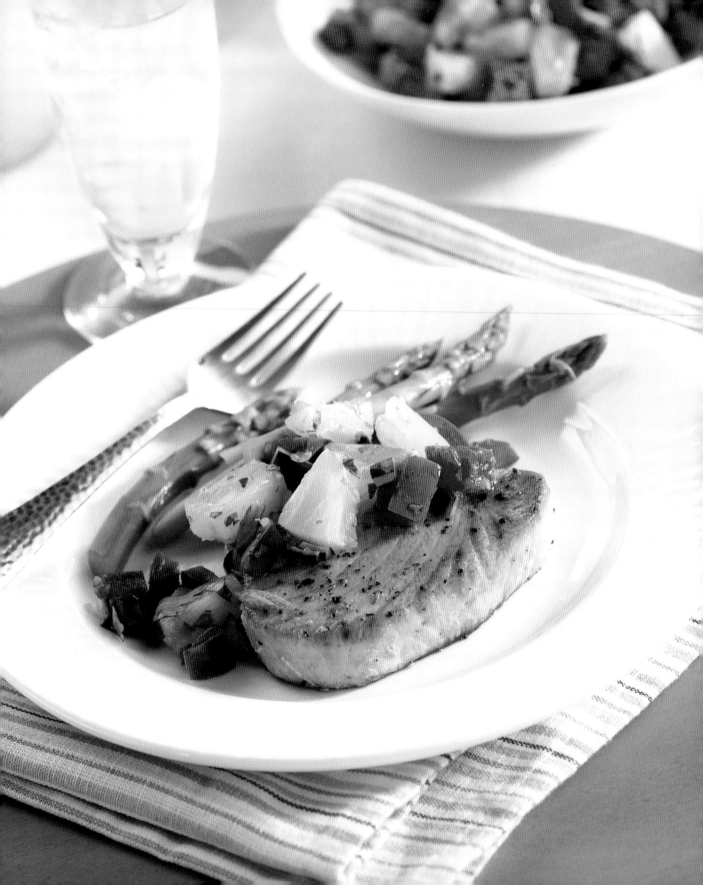

BUDDHA'S DELIGHT

1 package (1 ounce) dried shiitake mushrooms
1 package (about 12 ounces) firm tofu, drained
1 tablespoon peanut or vegetable oil
2 cups diagonally cut 1-inch asparagus pieces
1 medium onion, cut into thin wedges
2 cloves garlic, minced
½ cup vegetable broth
3 tablespoons hoisin sauce
¼ cup coarsely chopped fresh cilantro or thinly sliced green onions

1. Place mushrooms in small bowl; cover with warm water. Let stand 20 minutes or until softened. Drain over fine-mesh strainer, squeezing out excess water into measuring cup; reserve liquid. Discard mushroom stems; slice caps.

2. Meanwhile, place tofu on plate or cutting board lined with paper towels; cover with more paper towels and place flat, heavy object on top. Press for 15 minutes. Cut tofu into ¾-inch cubes or triangles.

3. Heat oil in wok or large skillet over medium-high heat. Add asparagus, onion and garlic; cook and stir 4 minutes. Add mushrooms, ¼ cup reserved mushroom liquid, broth and hoisin sauce. Reduce heat to medium-low. Simmer, uncovered, 2 to 3 minutes or until asparagus is crisp-tender. Add tofu; cook and stir until heated through.

4. Ladle mixture into serving bowls; sprinkle with cilantro.   *Makes 2 servings*

Nutrients per Serving: *½ of total recipe*
Calories: 332, **Calories from Fat:** 38%, **Total Fat:** 15g,
Saturated Fat: 3g, **Cholesterol:** <1mg, **Sodium:** 553mg,
Carbohydrate: 36g, **Fiber:** 8g, **Protein:** 20g

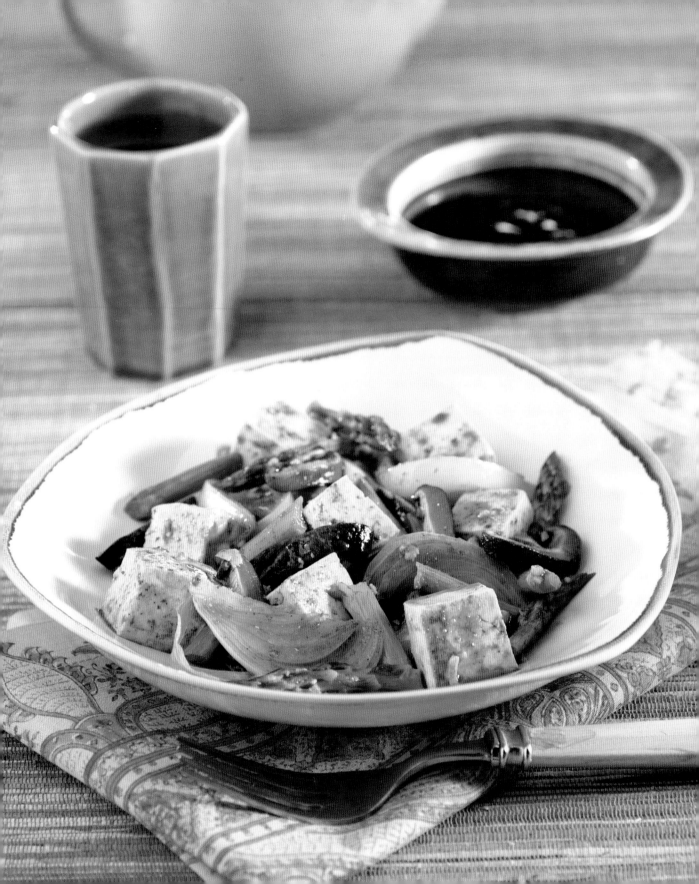

SEARED PORK ROAST WITH CURRANT CHERRY SALSA

1½ teaspoons chili powder

¾ teaspoon salt

½ teaspoon garlic powder

½ teaspoon paprika

¼ teaspoon ground allspice

1 boneless pork loin roast (2 pounds)

Nonstick cooking spray

½ cup water

1 pound bag frozen pitted dark cherries, thawed, drained and halved

¼ cup currants or dark raisins

1 teaspoon grated orange peel

1 teaspoon balsamic vinegar

⅛ teaspoon red pepper flakes

Slow Cooker Directions

1. Combine chili powder, salt, garlic powder, paprika and allspice in small bowl; coat pork with spices. Spray large nonstick skillet with cooking spray; heat over medium-high heat. Brown roast on all sides. Place in slow cooker. Pour water into skillet, stirring to scrape up browned bits; pour into slow cooker. Cover; cook on LOW 6 to 8 hours.

2. Remove pork from slow cooker. Tent with foil; keep warm. Strain juices from slow cooker; discard solids. Pour juice into small saucepan; keep warm over low heat.

3. Turn slow cooker to HIGH. Add cherries, currants, orange peel, vinegar and red pepper flakes. Cover; cook 30 minutes. Slice pork and arrange on serving platter. Spoon warm juices over meat. Serve with salsa. *Makes 8 servings*

Nutrients per Serving: *⅛ of total recipe*
Calories: 217, **Calories from Fat:** 38%, **Total Fat:** 9g,
Saturated Fat: 3g, **Cholesterol:** 72mg, **Sodium:** 300mg,
Carbohydrate: 10g, **Fiber:** 1g, **Protein:** 23g

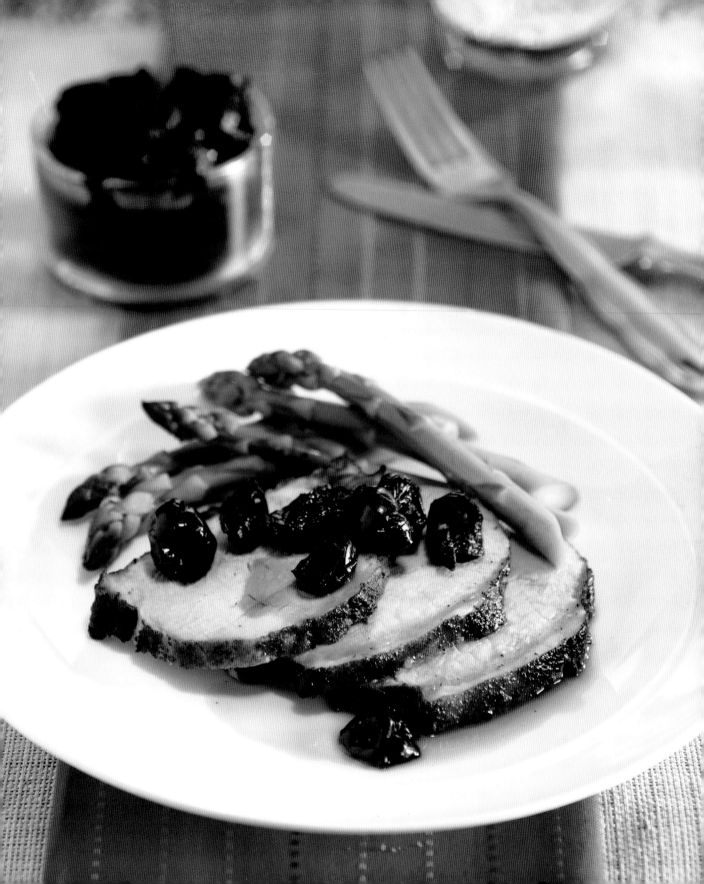

BOLOGNESE SAUCE & PENNE PASTA

     8 ounces 95% lean ground beef
⅓ cup chopped onion
     1 clove garlic, minced
     1 can (8 ounces) tomato sauce
⅓ cup chopped carrot
¼ cup water
     2 tablespoons red wine
     1 teaspoon Italian seasoning
1½ cups hot cooked penne pasta
     Chopped fresh parsley

1. Brown beef, onion and garlic 6 to 8 minutes in medium saucepan over medium-high heat, stirring to break up meat. Drain fat. Add tomato sauce, carrot, water, wine and Italian seasoning; bring to a boil. Reduce heat; simmer 15 minutes.

2. Serve sauce over pasta. Sprinkle with parsley.   *Makes 2 servings*

Nutrients per Serving: *¾ cup cooked pasta*
with about ½ of sauce
Calories: 292, **Calories from Fat:** 14%, **Total Fat:** 5g,
Saturated Fat: 2g, **Cholesterol:** 45mg, **Sodium:** 734mg,
Carbohydrate: 40g, **Fiber:** 4g, **Protein:** 21g

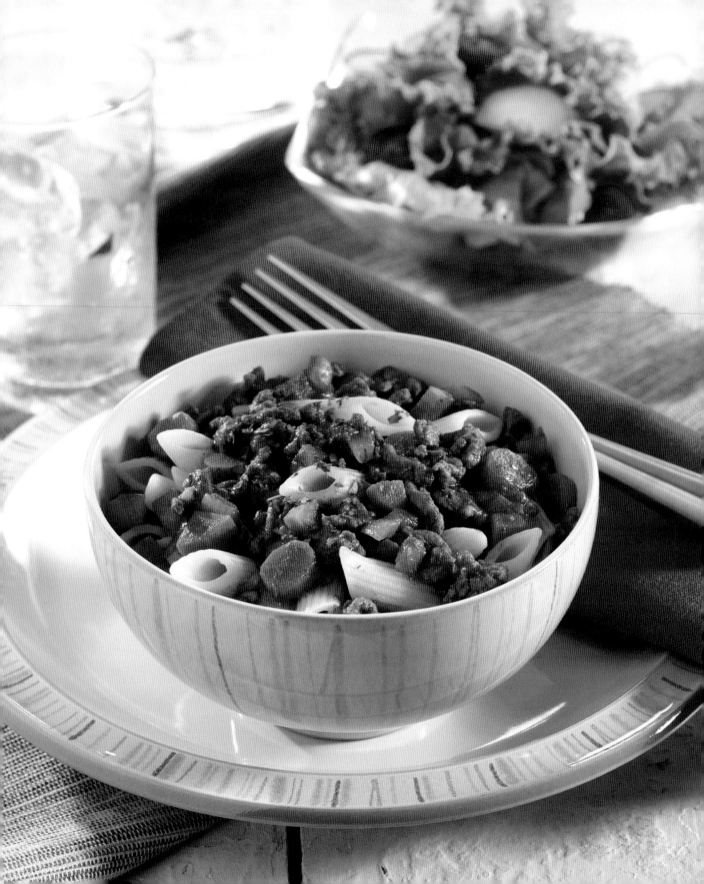

GREEK-STYLE SALMON

1½ teaspoons olive oil

1¾ cups diced tomatoes, drained

6 pitted black olives, coarsely chopped

4 pitted green olives, coarsely chopped

3 tablespoons lemon juice

2 tablespoons chopped fresh Italian parsley

1 tablespoon capers, rinsed and drained

2 cloves garlic, thinly sliced

¼ teaspoon black pepper

1 pound salmon fillets

1. Heat oil in large nonstick skillet over medium heat. Add tomatoes, olives, lemon juice, parsley, capers, garlic and pepper. Bring to a simmer, stirring frequently. Simmer 5 minutes or until reduced by about one third, stirring occasionally.

2. Rinse salmon and pat dry with paper towels. Push sauce to one side of skillet. Add salmon; spoon sauce over salmon. Cover and cook 10 to 15 minutes or until salmon begins to flake when tested with fork.

Makes 4 servings

Nutrients per Serving: *4 ounces fish with about ½ cup sauce*
Calories: 254, **Calories from Fat:** 52%, **Total Fat:** 15g,
Saturated Fat: 3g, **Cholesterol:** 66mg, **Sodium:** 196mg,
Carbohydrate: 6g, **Fiber:** 2g, **Protein:** 24g

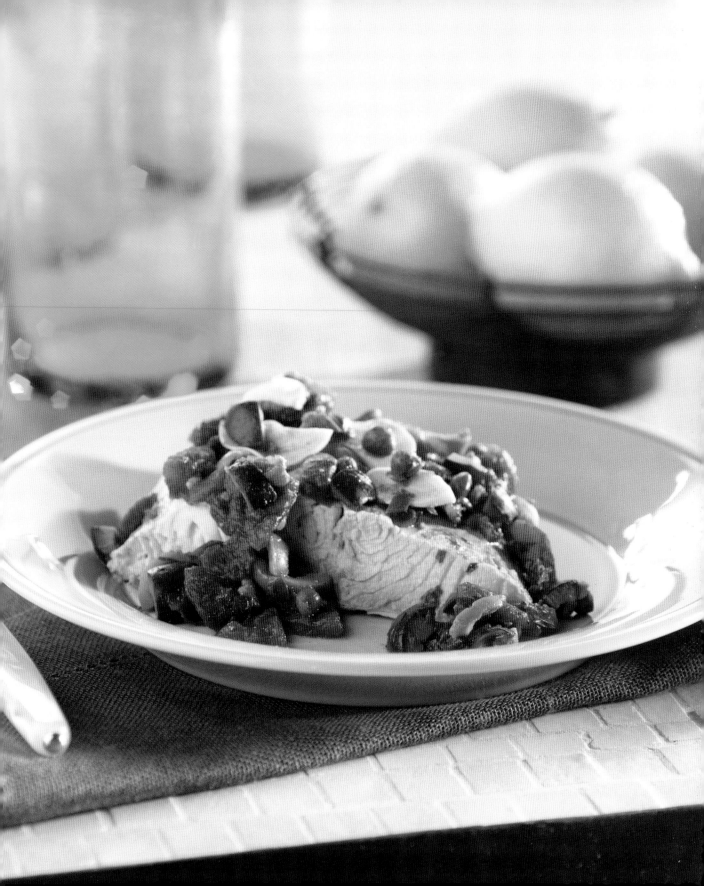

FIESTA BEEF ENCHILADAS

   1 pound 95% lean ground beef

   ½ cup sliced green onions

   2 teaspoons minced garlic

1½ cups chopped tomatoes, divided

   1 cup cooked white or brown rice

   1 cup (4 ounces) shredded reduced-fat Mexican cheese blend
        or Cheddar cheese, divided

   ¾ cup frozen corn, thawed

   ½ cup salsa or picante sauce

 12 (6- to 7-inch) corn tortillas

   1 can (10 ounces) enchilada sauce

   1 cup shredded romaine lettuce

1. Preheat oven to 375°F. Spray 13×9-inch baking dish with nonstick cooking spray.

2. Brown beef 6 to 8 minutes in medium nonstick skillet over medium-high heat, stirring to break up meat. Drain fat. Add green onions and garlic; cook and stir 2 minutes. Remove from heat.

3. Stir 1 cup tomatoes, rice, ½ cup cheese, corn and salsa into meat mixture. Spoon mixture evenly down center of tortillas. Roll up to enclose fillings; place seam side down in prepared dish. Spoon enchilada sauce evenly over enchiladas. Cover with foil.

4. Bake 20 minutes or until heated through. Sprinkle with remaining ½ cup cheese; bake 5 minutes or until cheese is melted. Top with lettuce and remaining ½ cup tomatoes just before serving. *Makes 6 servings*

Nutrients per Serving: *2 enchiladas*
Calories: 341, **Calories from Fat:** 30%, **Total Fat:** 11g,
Saturated Fat: 5g, **Cholesterol:** 38mg, **Sodium:** 465mg,
Carbohydrate: 43g, **Fiber:** 4g, **Protein:** 17g

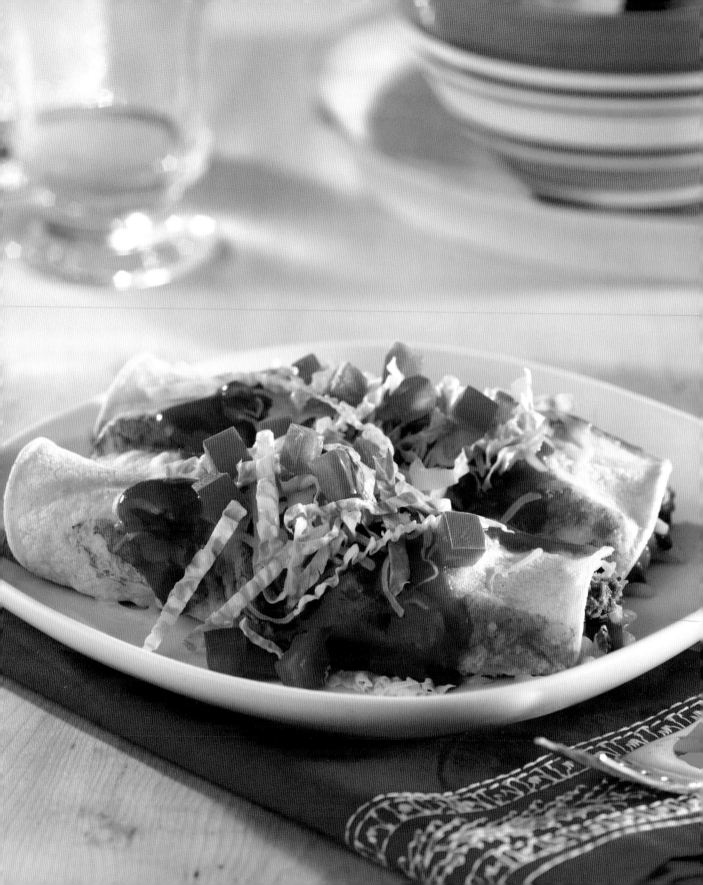

CHICKEN GOULASH

1 small onion, chopped

1 stalk celery, chopped

1 medium carrot, chopped

1 clove garlic, minced

½ cup reduced-sodium chicken broth

½ cup no-salt-added tomato purée

1 teaspoon paprika

¼ teaspoon dried marjoram or oregano

⅛ teaspoon black pepper

5 ounces boneless skinless chicken thighs, trimmed

1 small unpeeled new potato, diced

1 heaping teaspoon all-purpose flour

¼ teaspoon salt (optional)

Slow Cooker Directions

1. Combine onion, celery, carrot and garlic in slow cooker. Whisk broth, tomato purée, paprika, marjoram and pepper in small bowl until well blended; pour over vegetables. Add chicken and potato. Cover; cook on LOW 5 to 6 hours.

2. Whisk flour into 2 tablespoons cooking liquid from slow cooker in small bowl until smooth and well blended. Stir flour mixture into slow cooker. Cover; cook on LOW 10 minutes. Stir in salt, if desired. *Makes 2 servings*

Nutrients per Serving: *1¼ cups*
Calories: 226, **Calories from Fat:** 13%, **Total Fat:** 3g,
Saturated Fat: <1g, **Cholesterol:** 60mg, **Sodium:** 156mg,
Carbohydrate: 31g, **Fiber:** 5g, **Protein:** 19g

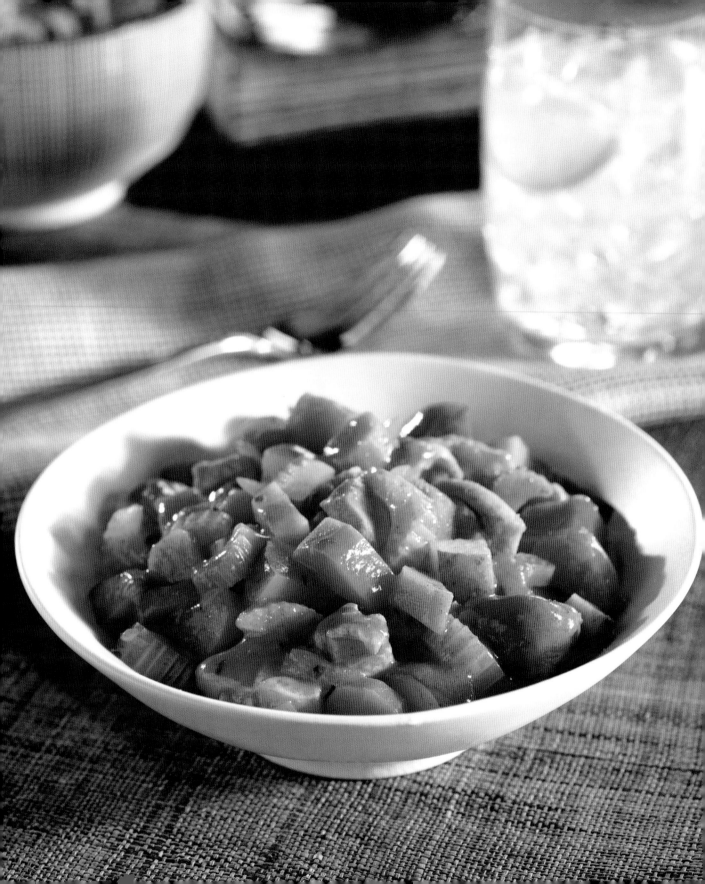

ITALIAN-STYLE MEATLOAF

1 can (6 ounces) no-salt-added tomato paste
½ cup water
½ cup dry red wine
1 teaspoon minced garlic
½ teaspoon dried basil
½ teaspoon dried oregano
¼ teaspoon salt
¾ pound 95% lean ground beef
¾ pound 93% lean ground turkey breast
1 cup fresh whole wheat bread crumbs (about 2 slices whole wheat bread)
½ cup shredded zucchini
¼ cup cholesterol-free egg substitute *or* 2 egg whites

1. Preheat oven to 350°F. Combine tomato paste, water, wine, garlic, basil, oregano and salt in small saucepan. Bring to a boil; reduce heat to low. Simmer, uncovered, 15 minutes.

2. Combine beef, turkey, bread crumbs, zucchini, egg substitute and ½ cup tomato mixture in large bowl; mix well. Shape into loaf; place in ungreased 9×5-inch loaf pan.

3. Bake 45 minutes. Drain fat. Spread remaining tomato mixture over meatloaf. Bake 15 minutes or until cooked through (160°F). Place on serving platter; let stand 10 minutes before slicing and serving. *Makes 8 servings*

Nutrients per Serving: *1 slice*
Calories: 187, **Calories from Fat:** 11%, **Total Fat:** 6g,
Saturated Fat: 2g, **Cholesterol:** 56mg, **Sodium:** 212mg,
Carbohydrate: 12g, **Fiber:** 2g, **Protein:** 19g

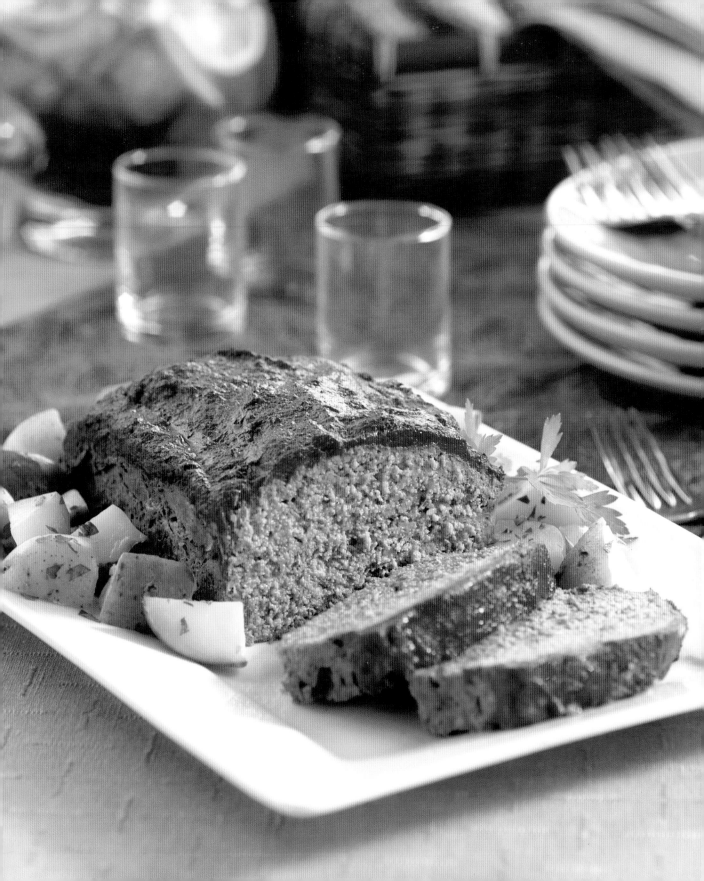

CUBAN GARLIC & LIME PORK CHOPS

4 boneless pork top loin chops, ¾ inch thick (about 1½ pounds)

2 tablespoons olive oil

2 tablespoons lime juice

2 tablespoons orange juice

2 teaspoons minced garlic

½ teaspoon salt, divided

½ teaspoon red pepper flakes

Salsa

2 small seedless oranges, peeled and chopped

1 medium cucumber, peeled, seeded and chopped

2 tablespoons chopped onion

2 tablespoons chopped fresh cilantro

1. Place pork chops in large resealable food storage bag. Add oil, lime juice, orange juice, garlic, ¼ teaspoon salt and red pepper flakes. Seal bag; turn to coat evenly. Marinate in refrigerator at least 1 hour or up to 24 hours.

2. Meanwhile, combine oranges, cucumber, onion and cilantro in small bowl; gently toss. Cover and refrigerate 1 hour or overnight.

3. Prepare grill for direct cooking. Remove pork chops from marinade; discard marinade. Grill or broil pork chops over medium-high heat 6 to 8 minutes per side or until no longer pink in center.

4. Sprinkle pork chops with remaining ¼ teaspoon salt just before serving. Serve with salsa.

Makes 2 servings

Nutrients per Serving: *1 pork chop with about ½ cup salsa*
Calories: 307, **Calories from Fat:** 33%, **Total Fat:** 11g,
Saturated Fat: 2g, **Cholesterol:** 94mg, **Sodium:** 610mg,
Carbohydrate: 12g, **Fiber:** 3g, **Protein:** 39g

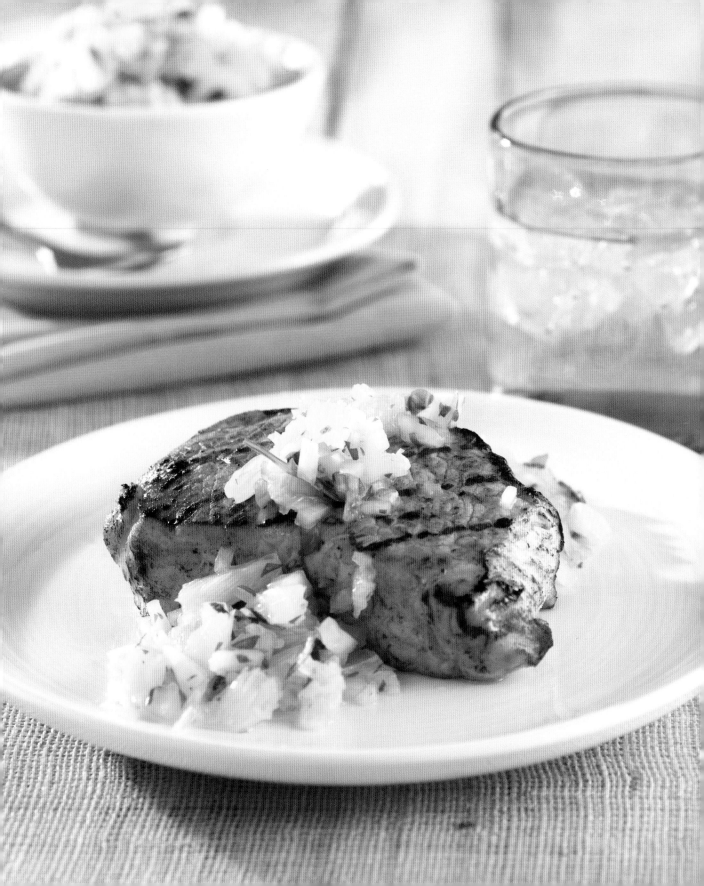

SAUSAGE & SHRIMP JAMBALAYA

1 teaspoon olive oil
1 cup chopped onion
1 large green bell pepper, cut into ¾-inch pieces
2 cloves garlic, minced
1¼ cups reduced-sodium chicken broth
1 can (about 14 ounces) diced tomatoes
⅔ cup uncooked rice
1 teaspoon dried thyme
½ teaspoon paprika
¼ teaspoon black pepper
8 ounces frozen medium cooked peeled shrimp
3 ounces kielbasa sausage, cut in half lengthwise, then into ¼-inch slices

1. Heat oil in large nonstick skillet over medium heat. Add onion and bell pepper; cook and stir 4 to 5 minutes. Add garlic; cook and stir 30 seconds. Add broth, tomatoes, rice, thyme, paprika and black pepper; bring to a boil. Reduce heat to low; cover and simmer 15 minutes.

2. Stir in shrimp and sausage; cover and simmer 5 minutes or until shrimp are heated through and rice is tender.
Makes 5 servings

Nutrients per Serving: *1¼ cups*
Calories: 210, **Calories from Fat:** 13%, **Total Fat:** 3g,
Saturated Fat: <1g, **Cholesterol:** 102mg, **Sodium:** 553mg,
Carbohydrate: 28g, **Fiber:** 2g, **Protein:** 17g

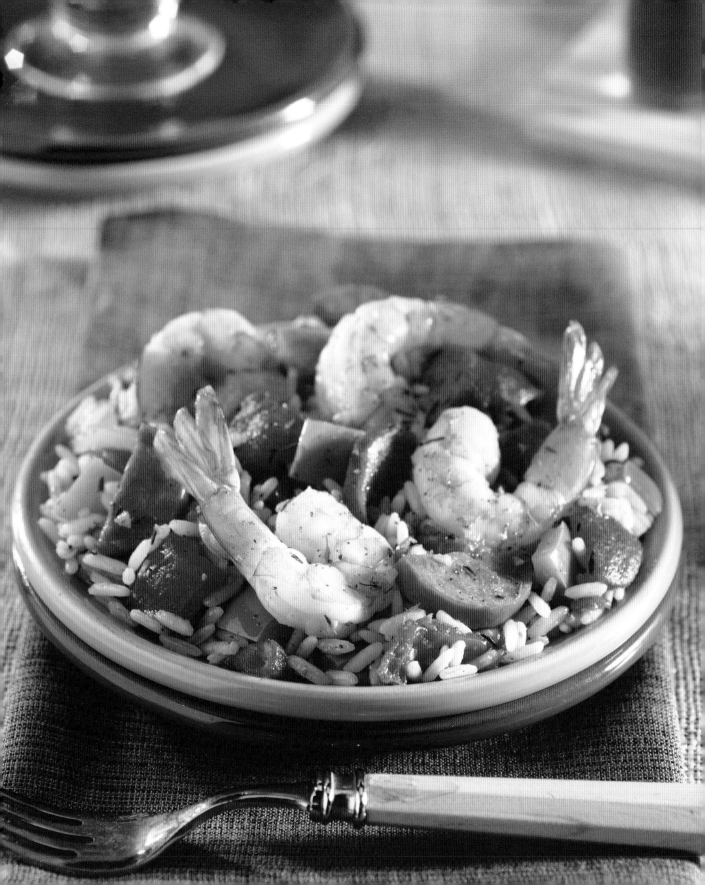

TUSCAN TURKEY AND WHITE BEAN SKILLET

1 teaspoon dried rosemary, divided

½ teaspoon garlic salt

½ teaspoon black pepper, divided

1 pound turkey breast cutlets, pounded to ¼-inch thickness

2 teaspoons canola oil, divided

1 can (about 15 ounces) no-salt-added navy beans or Great Northern beans, rinsed and drained

1 can (about 14 ounces) fire-roasted diced tomatoes

¼ cup grated Parmesan cheese

1. Combine ½ teaspoon rosemary, garlic salt and ¼ teaspoon pepper in small bowl; mix well. Sprinkle over turkey.

2. Heat 1 teaspoon oil in large nonstick skillet over medium heat. Add half of turkey; cook 2 to 3 minutes per side or until cooked through (165°F). Transfer to large platter; tent with foil to keep warm. Repeat with remaining 1 teaspoon oil and half of turkey.

3. Add beans, tomatoes, remaining ½ teaspoon rosemary and ¼ teaspoon pepper to same skillet. Bring to a boil over high heat. Reduce heat; simmer 5 minutes.

4. Spoon bean mixture over and around turkey. Sprinkle with cheese.

Makes 6 servings

Nutrients per Serving: *1 cup*
Calories: 230, **Calories from Fat:** 16%, **Total Fat:** 4g,
Saturated Fat: 1g, **Cholesterol:** 36mg, **Sodium:** 334mg,
Carbohydrate: 23g, **Fiber:** 9g, **Protein:** 25g

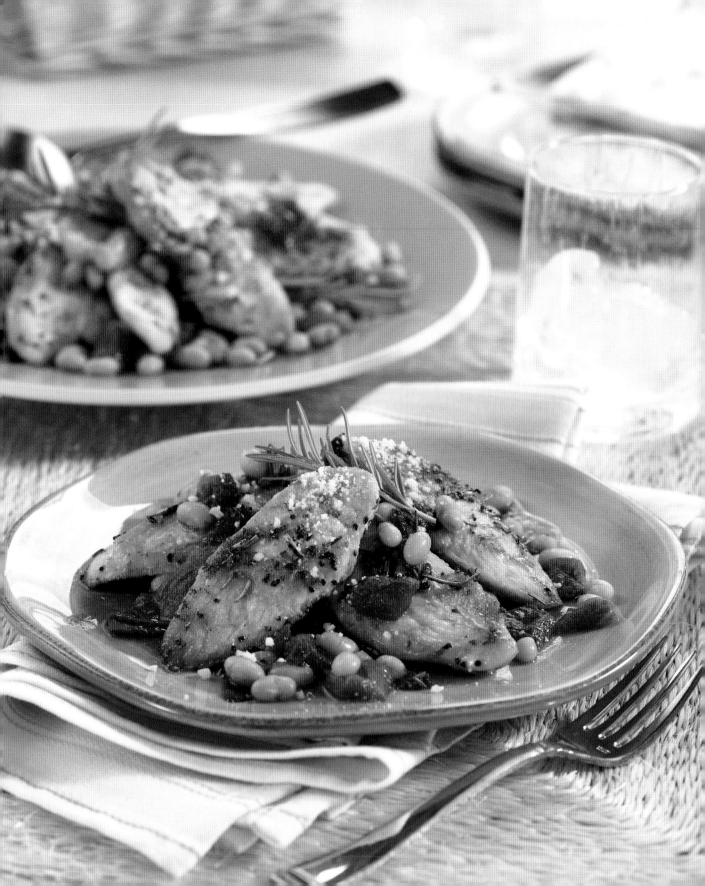

SIDE DISHES

BEETS IN SPICY MUSTARD SAUCE

   3 pounds beets, trimmed
¼ cup reduced-fat sour cream
   2 tablespoons spicy brown mustard
   2 teaspoons lemon juice
   2 cloves garlic, minced
¼ teaspoon black pepper
⅛ teaspoon dried thyme

1. Place beets in large saucepan; add enough water to cover by 1 inch. Bring to a boil over medium-high heat. Reduce heat to medium-low; cover and simmer 25 minutes or until tender. Drain. Peel beets; cut into ¼-inch-thick slices.

2. Combine sour cream, mustard, lemon juice, garlic, pepper and thyme in small saucepan; cook and stir over medium heat until heated through. Spoon sauce over beets; gently toss to coat.

Makes 4 servings

Nutrients per Serving: *¼ of total recipe*
Calories: 116, **Calories from Fat:** 16%, **Total Fat:** 2g,
Saturated Fat: 0g, **Cholesterol:** 6mg, **Sodium:** 253mg,
Carbohydrate: 21g, **Fiber:** 6g, **Protein:** 4g

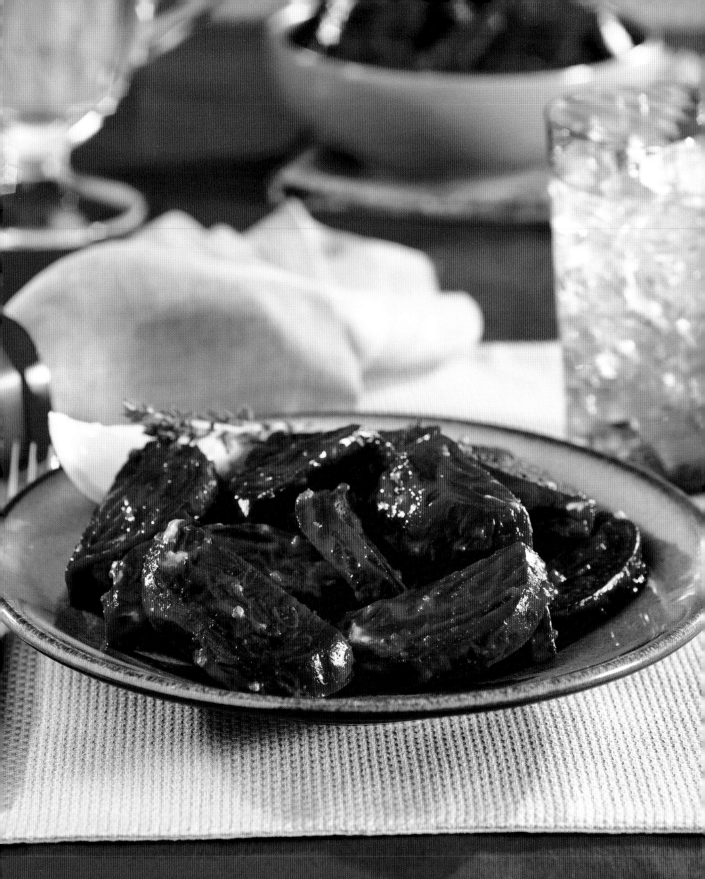

BULGUR WITH ASPARAGUS AND SPRING HERBS

⅔ cup uncooked bulgur

2 cups sliced asparagus (1-inch pieces)

½ cup frozen peas, thawed

⅔ cup chopped fresh Italian parsley

2 teaspoons finely chopped fresh mint

3 tablespoons lemon juice

1 tablespoon orange juice

1 tablespoon extra virgin olive oil

⅛ teaspoon salt

⅛ teaspoon black pepper

1. Prepare bulgur according to package directions. Drain. Cool completely.

2. Steam asparagus in steamer basket over boiling water 3 to 4 minutes or until bright green and crisp-tender. Cool under cold running water; drain and pat dry with paper towels.

3. Combine bulgur, asparagus, peas, parsley and mint in large bowl. Whisk lemon juice, orange juice, oil, salt and pepper in small bowl until well blended. Pour over bulgur mixture; gently toss.

Makes 4 servings

Nutrients per Serving: *1 cup*
Calories: 148, **Calories from Fat:** 24%, **Total Fat:** 4g,
Saturated Fat: 1g, **Cholesterol:** 0mg, **Sodium:** 98mg,
Carbohydrate: 25g, **Fiber:** 7g, **Protein:** 6g

Note: Bulgur is a whole grain that's high in fiber and protein. It's also a good source of iron, magnesium and B vitamins.

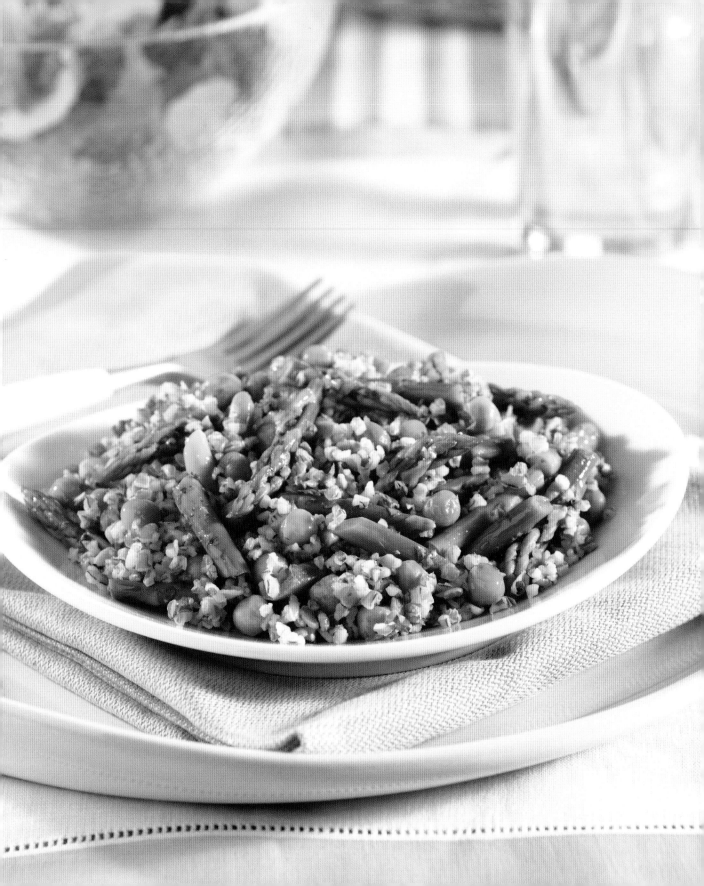

CONFETTI BLACK BEANS

1 cup dried black beans

3 cups water

1 can (about 14 ounces) reduced-sodium chicken broth

1 bay leaf

1½ teaspoons olive oil

1 medium onion, chopped

¼ cup chopped red bell pepper

¼ cup chopped yellow bell pepper

2 cloves garlic, minced

1 jalapeño pepper,* finely chopped

1 large tomato, seeded and chopped

½ teaspoon salt

⅛ teaspoon black pepper

Hot pepper sauce (optional)

Jalapeño peppers can sting and irritate the skin, so wear rubber gloves when handling peppers and do not touch your eyes.

1. Sort and rinse beans; cover with water. Soak 8 hours or overnight. Drain.

2. Combine beans and broth in large saucepan; bring to a boil over high heat. Add bay leaf. Reduce heat to low; cover and simmer 1½ hours or until beans are tender.

3. Heat oil in large nonstick skillet over medium heat. Add onion, bell peppers, garlic and jalapeño; cook and stir 8 to 10 minutes or until onion is translucent. Add tomato, salt and black pepper; cook 5 minutes.

4. Add onion mixture to beans; cook 15 to 20 minutes. Remove and discard bay leaf. Serve with hot pepper sauce, if desired. *Makes 6 servings*

Nutrients per Serving: *½ cup*
Calories: 146, **Calories from Fat:** 14%, **Total Fat:** 2g,
Saturated Fat: <1g, **Cholesterol:** 0mg, **Sodium:** 209mg,
Carbohydrate: 24g, **Fiber:** 6g, **Protein:** 8g

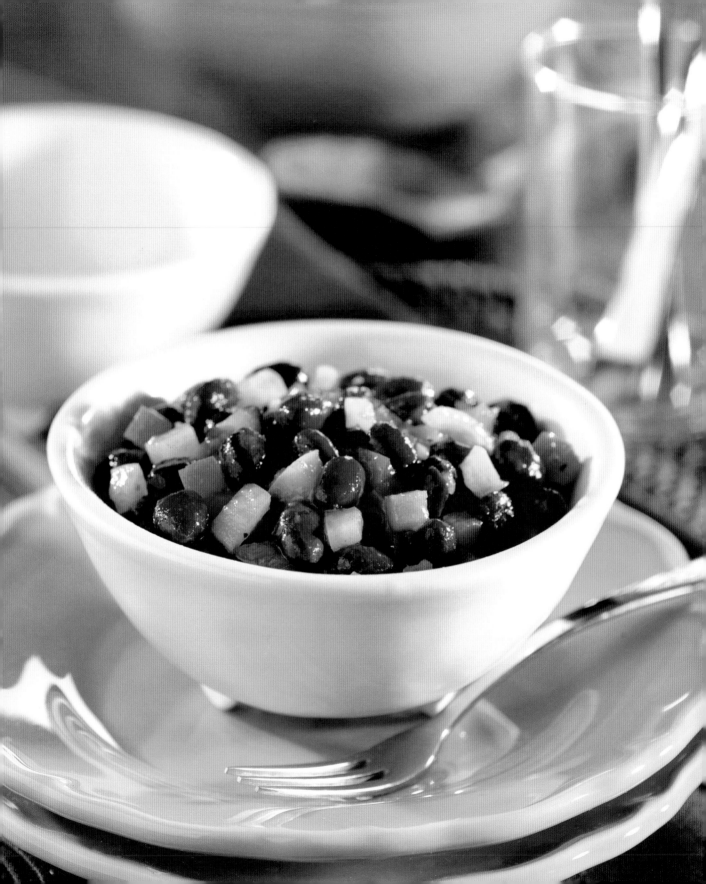

BUTTERNUT SQUASH WITH APPLES, CRANBERRIES AND WALNUTS

2 teaspoons butter

3 cups cubed (about ½ inch) butternut squash

1 tablespoon packed brown sugar

¼ teaspoon ground cinnamon

¼ teaspoon salt

⅛ teaspoon black pepper

1 cup water

1 cup cubed (about ½ inch) peeled Granny Smith apple

2 tablespoons dried cranberries

2 tablespoons chopped walnuts

1. Melt butter in large nonstick skillet over medium heat. Add squash, gently stirring to coat. Add brown sugar, cinnamon, salt and pepper; gently stir. Add water; cover and bring to a simmer.

2. Reduce heat to low; simmer 10 minutes. Stir in apple and cranberries. Cover and simmer 10 minutes or until squash is tender. Stir in walnuts just before serving.

Makes 4 servings

Nutrients per Serving: *¾ cup*
Calories: 129, **Calories from Fat:** 28%, **Total Fat:** 4g,
Saturated Fat: 1g, **Cholesterol:** 5mg, **Sodium:** 170mg,
Carbohydrate: 23g, **Fiber:** 3g, **Protein:** 2g

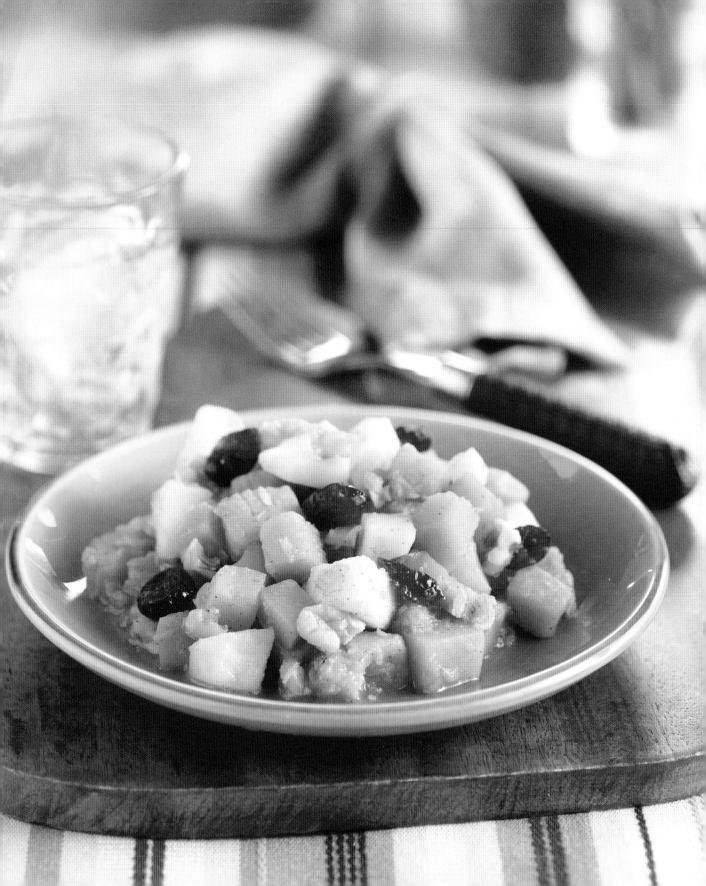

OVEN "FRIES"

2 small russet potatoes (10 ounces), refrigerated (see Note)
2 teaspoons olive oil
¼ teaspoon salt or onion salt

1. Preheat oven to 450°F. Peel potatoes and cut lengthwise into ¼-inch strips. Place in colander; rinse under cold running water 2 minutes. Drain. Pat dry with paper towels.

2. Place potatoes in large resealable food storage bag. Drizzle with oil. Seal bag; turn to coat evenly. Arrange potatoes in single layer on baking sheet

3. Bake 20 to 25 minutes or until light brown and crisp. Sprinkle with salt.

Makes 2 servings

Nutrients per Serving: *½ of fries*
Calories: 237, **Calories from Fat:** 26%, **Total Fat:** 7g,
Saturated Fat: 1g, **Cholesterol:** 0mg, **Sodium:** 300mg,
Carbohydrate: 41g, **Fiber:** 3g, **Protein:** 4g

Note: Refrigerating potatoes—usually not recommended for storage—converts the starch in the potatoes to sugar, which enhances the browning when the potatoes are baked. Do not refrigerate the potatoes longer than 2 days, because they may develop a sweet flavor.

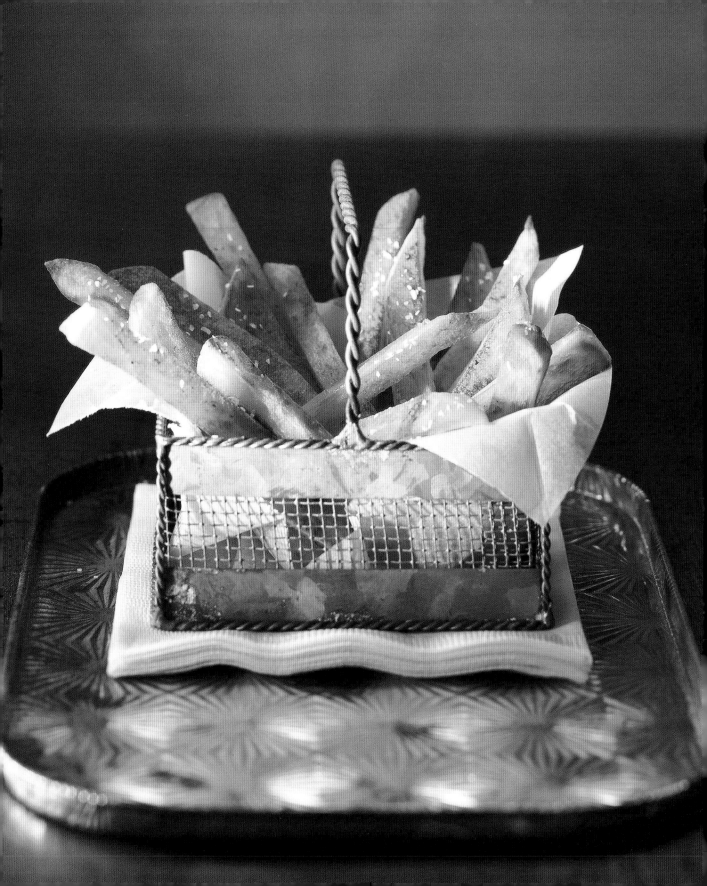

BRUSSELS SPROUTS IN ORANGE SAUCE

4 cups fresh Brussels sprouts

1 can (6 ounces) unsweetened orange juice

½ cup water

1 teaspoon shredded or grated orange peel (optional)

½ teaspoon cornstarch

¼ teaspoon red pepper flakes (optional)

¼ teaspoon ground cinnamon

Salt and black pepper

1. Combine Brussels sprouts, orange juice, water, orange peel, if desired, cornstarch, red pepper flakes, if desired, and cinnamon in medium saucepan. Cover and simmer 6 to 7 minutes or until sprouts are almost tender.

2. Uncover and simmer, stirring occasionally, until most of liquid has evaporated. Season with salt and pepper.

Makes 4 servings

Nutrients per Serving: *¼ of total recipe*
Calories: 59, **Calories from Fat:** 5%, **Total Fat:** <1g,
Saturated Fat: 0g, **Cholesterol:** 0mg, **Sodium:** 23mg,
Carbohydrate: 13g, **Fiber:** 4g, **Protein:** 3g

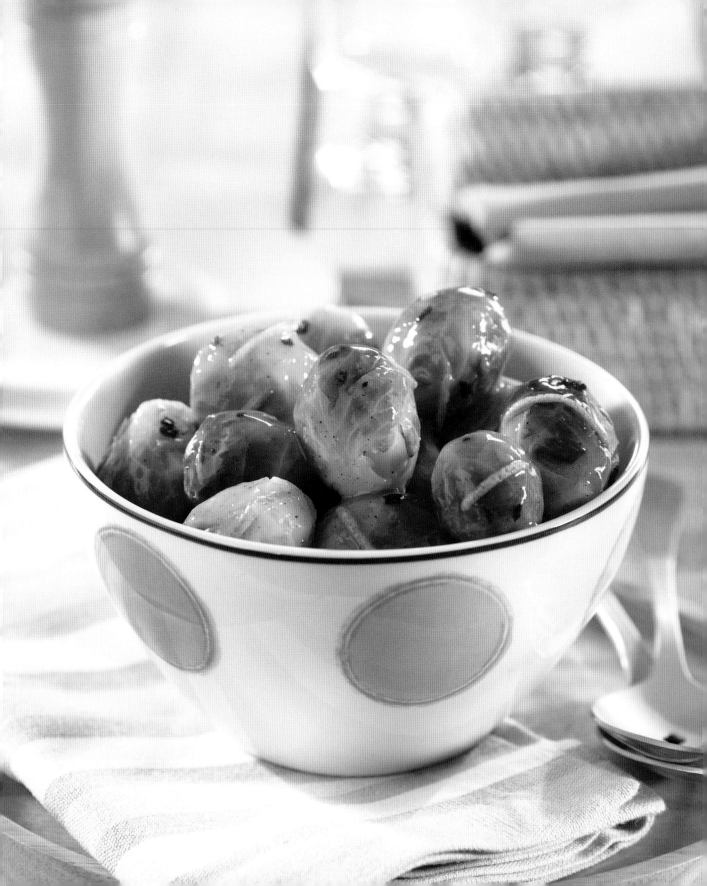

RATATOUILLE WITH PARMESAN CHEESE

Nonstick cooking spray
1 baby eggplant, diced, *or* 1 cup diced regular eggplant
2 medium tomatoes, chopped
1 small zucchini, diced
1 cup sliced mushrooms
½ cup no-salt-added tomato purée
1 large shallot *or* ½ small onion, chopped
1 clove garlic, minced
¾ teaspoon dried oregano
⅛ teaspoon dried rosemary
⅛ teaspoon black pepper
2 tablespoons shredded fresh basil
2 teaspoons lemon juice
¼ teaspoon salt (optional)
¼ cup shredded Parmesan cheese

Slow Cooker Directions

1. Spray large nonstick skillet with cooking spray. Add eggplant; cook and stir over medium-high heat 5 minutes or until lightly browned. Transfer to slow cooker.

2. Add tomatoes, zucchini, mushrooms, tomato purée, shallot, garlic, oregano, rosemary and pepper to slow cooker. Cover; cook on LOW 6 hours.

3. Stir in basil, lemon juice and salt, if desired. Turn off slow cooker; let stand 5 minutes.

4. Divide ratatouille evenly among four serving bowls. Top each serving with 1 tablespoon cheese.

Makes 4 servings

Nutrients per Serving: *½ cup*
Calories: 96, **Calories from Fat:** 16%, **Total Fat:** 2g,
Saturated Fat: 1g, **Cholesterol:** 4mg, **Sodium:** 98mg,
Carbohydrate: 17g, **Fiber:** 7g, **Protein:** 7g

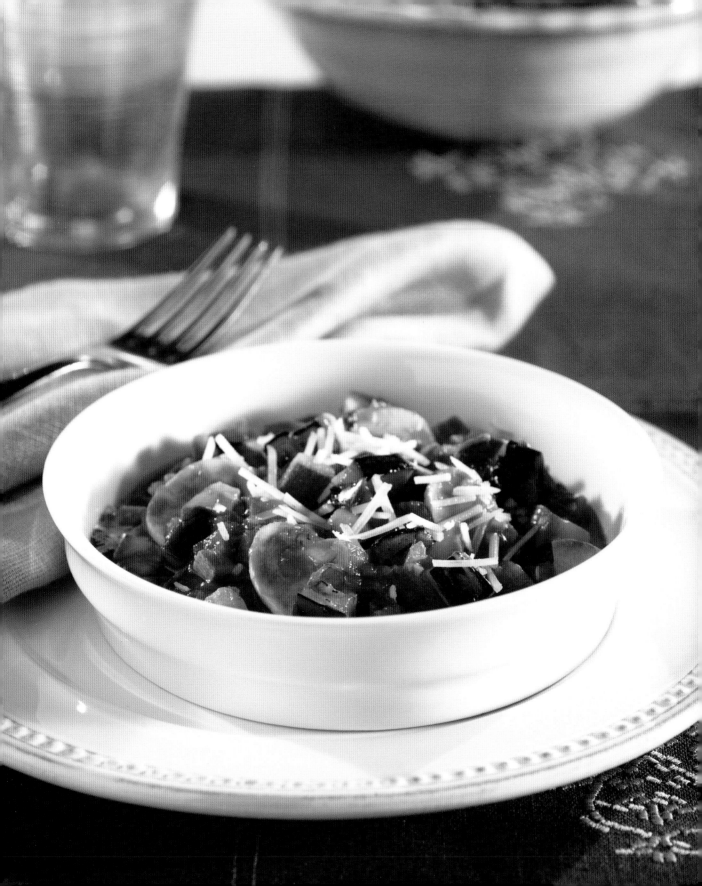

CHILE AND LIME QUINOA

½ cup quinoa

1 cup water

1 small jalapeño pepper,* minced

2 tablespoons finely chopped green onion

2 tablespoons olive oil

1 tablespoon fresh lime juice

¼ teaspoon salt

¼ teaspoon ground cumin

¼ teaspoon chili powder

⅛ teaspoon black pepper

Jalapeño peppers can sting and irritate the skin, so wear rubber gloves when handling peppers and do not touch your eyes.

1. Place quinoa in fine-mesh strainer; rinse well under cold running water. Combine quinoa and water in small saucepan; bring to a boil over high heat. Reduce heat to low; cover and simmer 12 to 15 minutes or until quinoa is tender. Drain. Cover; let stand 5 minutes.

2. Stir jalapeño, green onion, oil, lime juice, salt, cumin, chili powder and black pepper into quinoa. Fluff mixture with fork. Serve warm or at room temperature.

Makes 4 servings

Nutrients per Serving: *½ cup*
Calories: 144, **Calories from Fat:** 50%, **Total Fat:** 8g,
Saturated Fat: 1g, **Cholesterol:** 0mg, **Sodium:** 153mg,
Carbohydrate: 16g, **Fiber:** 2g, **Protein:** 3g

Note: Quinoa is a high-protein grain with a flavor similar to couscous. It cooks up more quickly than rice and has less carbohydrates than any other grain. Look for it in the rice and dried beans section or in the natural foods aisle of the supermarket.

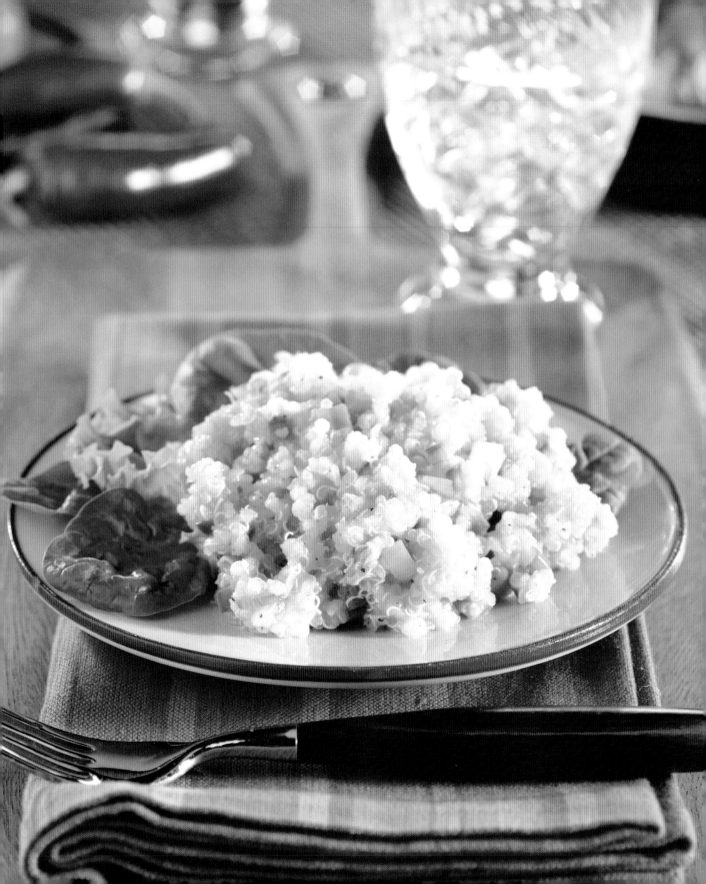

VEGETABLES AND SUN-DRIED TOMATOES

3 cups water

1 pound green beans

3 teaspoons olive oil, divided

5 ounces mushrooms, sliced

½ cup sliced almonds, toasted*

½ cup sun-dried tomatoes, sliced

¼ teaspoon salt

*To toast almonds, spread in single layer in heavy-bottomed skillet. Cook over medium heat 1 to 2 minutes, stirring frequently, until lightly browned. Remove from skillet immediately. Cool before using.

1. Bring water to a boil in medium saucepan. Add green beans; cook 4 minutes. Drain.

2. Heat 2 teaspoons oil in large skillet over medium heat. Add green beans, mushrooms and almonds; cook and stir 3 minutes. Add sun-dried tomatoes and remaining 1 teaspoon oil; cook and stir 2 to 3 minutes. Remove from heat.

3. Cover and let stand 15 minutes to allow flavors to develop. Season with salt.

Makes 6 servings

Nutrients per Serving: *⅔ cup*
Calories: 101, **Calories from Fat:** 53%, **Total Fat:** 6g,
Saturated Fat: 1g, **Cholesterol:** 0mg, **Sodium:** 193mg,
Carbohydrate: 11g, **Fiber:** 4g, **Protein:** 4g

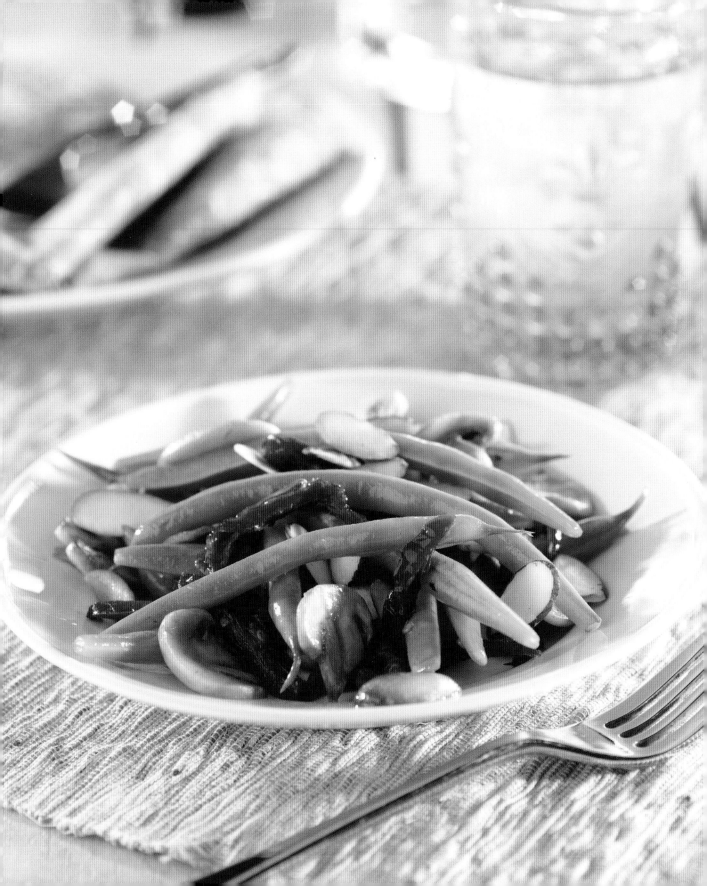

OLD-FASHIONED HERB STUFFING

6 slices (8 ounces) whole wheat, rye or white bread (or combination),
    cut into ½-inch cubes

1 tablespoon margarine or butter

1 cup chopped onion

½ cup thinly sliced celery

½ cup thinly sliced carrot

1 cup fat-free reduced-sodium chicken broth

1 tablespoon chopped fresh thyme *or* 1 teaspoon dried thyme

1 tablespoon chopped fresh sage *or* 1 teaspoon dried sage

½ teaspoon paprika

¼ teaspoon black pepper

1. Preheat oven to 350°F. Arrange bread cubes on baking sheet; bake 10 minutes or until dry.

2. Spray 1½-quart baking dish with nonstick cooking spray.

3. Melt margarine in large saucepan over medium heat. Add onion, celery and carrot; cook and stir 10 minutes or until vegetables are tender. Add broth, thyme, sage, paprika and pepper; bring to a simmer. Stir in bread cubes. Spoon into prepared dish.

4. Cover with foil; bake 25 to 30 minutes or until heated through.

Makes 4 servings

Nutrients per Serving: *¼ of total recipe*
Calories: 199, **Calories from Fat:** 23%, **Total Fat:** 5g,
Saturated Fat: 1g, **Cholesterol:** 0mg, **Sodium:** 395mg,
Carbohydrate: 32g, **Fiber:** 5g, **Protein:** 8g

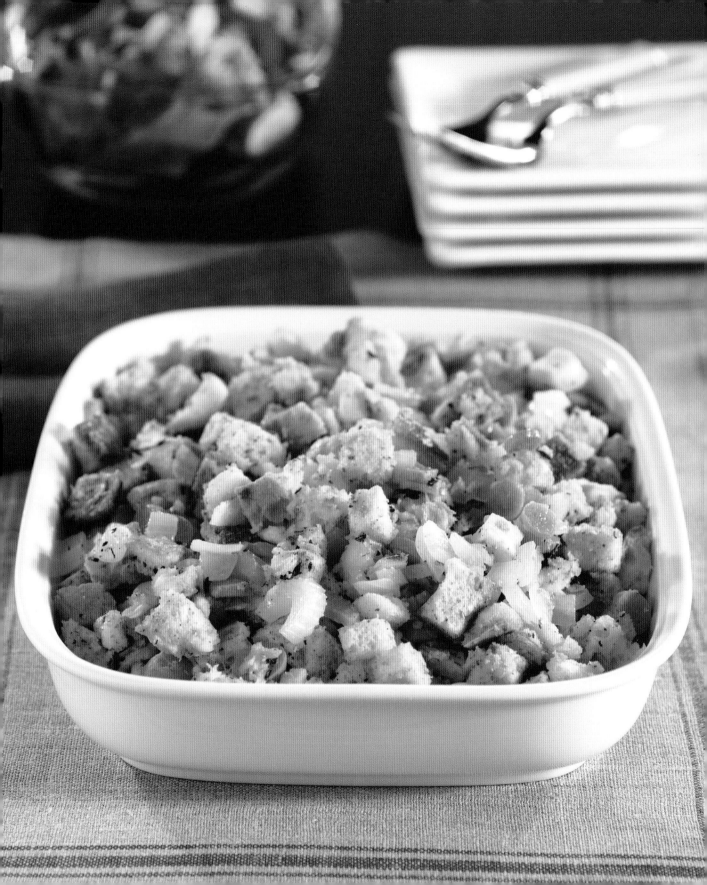

GARLICKY MUSTARD GREENS

2 pounds mustard greens

1 teaspoon olive oil

1 cup chopped onion

2 cloves garlic, minced

¾ cup chopped red bell pepper

½ cup fat-free reduced-sodium chicken or vegetable broth

1 tablespoon cider vinegar

1 teaspoon sugar

1. Remove stems and any wilted leaves from greens. Stack several leaves; roll up. Cut crosswise into 1-inch slices. Repeat with remaining greens.

2. Heat oil in large saucepan over medium heat. Add onion and garlic; cook and stir 5 minutes or until onion is tender. Stir in greens, bell pepper and broth. Reduce heat to low. Cover and cook 25 minutes or until greens are tender, stirring occasionally.

3. Whisk vinegar and sugar in small bowl until sugar is dissolved. Stir into cooked greens; remove from heat. Serve immediately.   *Makes 4 servings*

Nutrients per Serving: *¼ of total recipe*
Calories: 72, **Calories from Fat:** 25%, **Total Fat:** 2g,
Saturated Fat: <1g, **Cholesterol:** 0mg, **Sodium:** 42mg,
Carbohydrate: 11g, **Fiber:** 5g, **Protein:** 6g

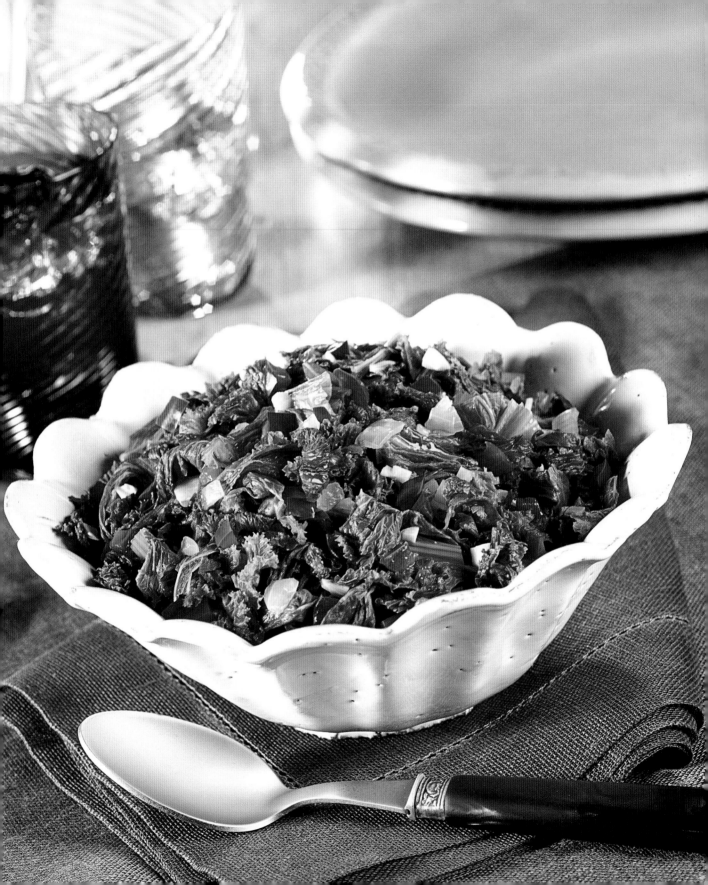

SWEET POTATO FRIES

1 large sweet potato (about 8 ounces)
2 teaspoons olive oil
¼ teaspoon salt (kosher or sea salt preferred)
¼ teaspoon black pepper
¼ teaspoon ground red pepper
   Sugar-free maple syrup (optional)

1. Preheat oven to 350°F. Spray baking sheet with nonstick cooking spray.

2. Peel sweet potato; cut lengthwise into long spears. Toss with oil, salt, black pepper and ground red pepper on prepared baking sheet. Arrange in single layer (spears should not touch).

3. Bake 45 minutes or until lightly browned. Serve with syrup for dipping, if desired.

Makes 2 servings

Nutrients per Serving: *½ of total recipe*
Calories: 139, **Calories from Fat:** 29%, **Total Fat:** 5g,
Saturated Fat: <1g, **Cholesterol:** 0mg, **Sodium:** 301mg,
Carbohydrate: 23g, **Fiber:** 4g, **Protein:** 2g

TIP   Kosher salt is pure sodium chloride, usually without any additives. It often comes in coarse crystals, giving a crunch and texture unlike that of table salt.

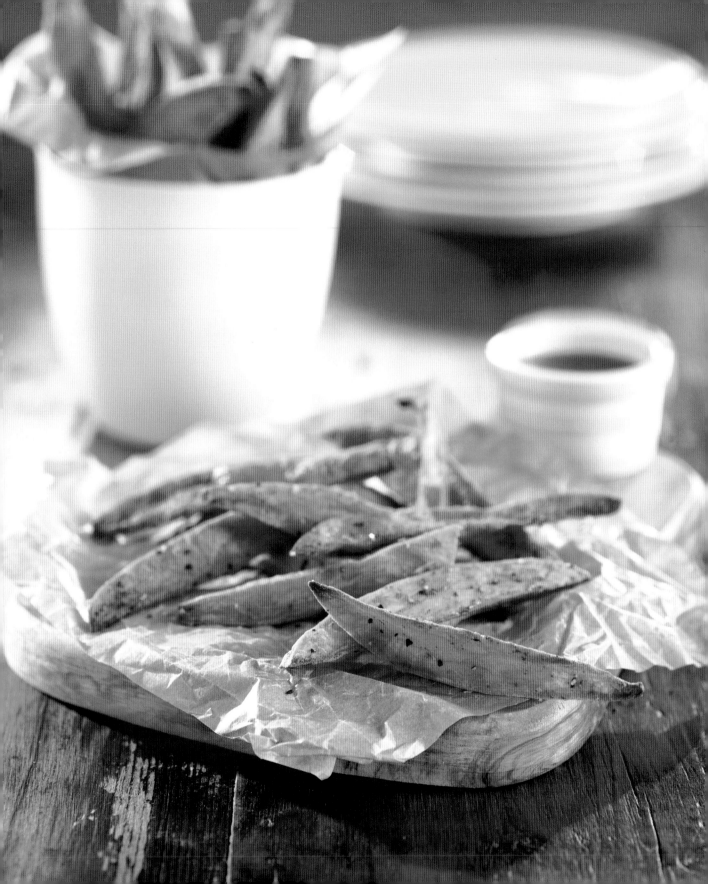

FAR EAST TABBOULEH

¾ cup uncooked bulgur
2 tablespoons lemon juice
2 tablespoons reduced-sodium teriyaki sauce
1 tablespoon olive oil
¾ cup diced seeded cucumber
¾ cup diced tomato
½ cup thinly sliced green onions
½ cup minced cilantro or parsley
1 tablespoon minced fresh ginger
1 clove garlic, minced

1. Prepare bulgur according to package directions. Drain.

2. Combine bulgur, lemon juice, teriyaki sauce and oil in large bowl. Stir in cucumber, tomato, green onions, cilantro, ginger and garlic until well combined. Cover and refrigerate 4 hours, stirring occasionally. *Makes 4 servings*

Nutrients per Serving: *¼ of total recipe*
Calories: 73, **Calories from Fat:** 23%, **Total Fat:** 2g,
Saturated Fat: <1g, **Cholesterol:** 0mg, **Sodium:** 156mg,
Carbohydrate: 13g, **Fiber:** 3g, **Protein:** 2g

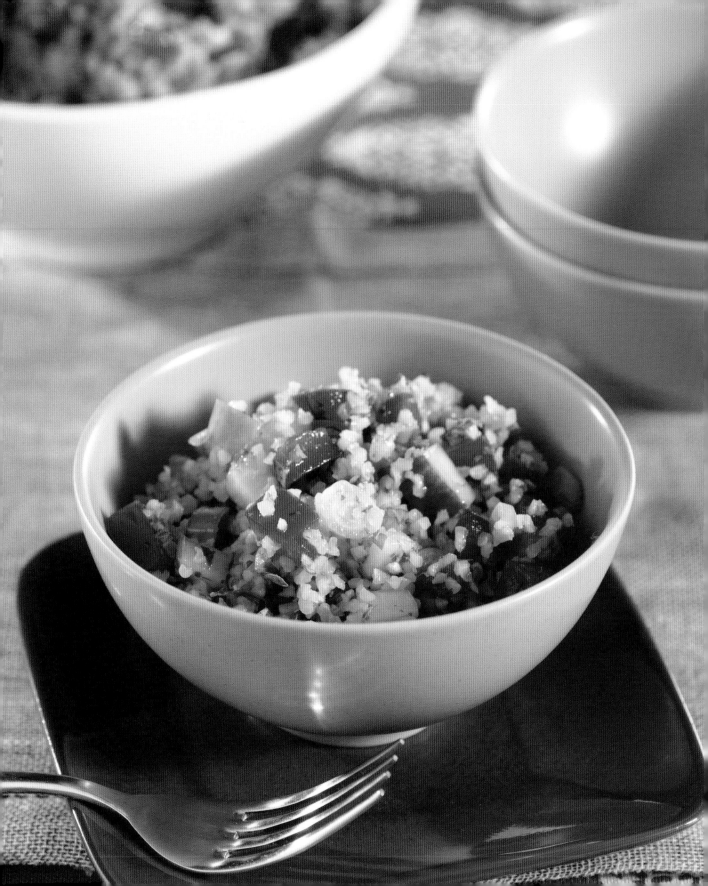

POTATO-ZUCCHINI PANCAKES

1 medium baking potato, unpeeled and shredded

½ small zucchini, shredded

1 green onion, thinly sliced, plus additional for garnish

1 egg white

2 tablespoons all-purpose flour

1 tablespoon vegetable oil

Sour cream (optional)

1. Combine potato, zucchini, 1 green onion, egg white and flour in medium bowl; mix well.

2. Heat oil in large nonstick skillet over medium heat. Pour ⅓ cupfuls potato mixture into skillet; flatten slightly. Cook 5 minutes per side or until browned.

3. Serve with sour cream, if desired. Garnish with additional green onion.

Makes 2 servings

Nutrients per Serving: *3 pancakes*
Calories: 190, **Calories from Fat:** 32%, **Total Fat:** 7g,
Saturated Fat: 1g, **Cholesterol:** 0mg, **Sodium:** 40mg,
Carbohydrate: 27g, **Fiber:** 2g, **Protein:** 6g

TIP   Save time by shredding both the potato and zucchini in a food processor fitted with a shredding disc. There's no need to wash the bowl in between because all the ingredients are mixed together before cooking.

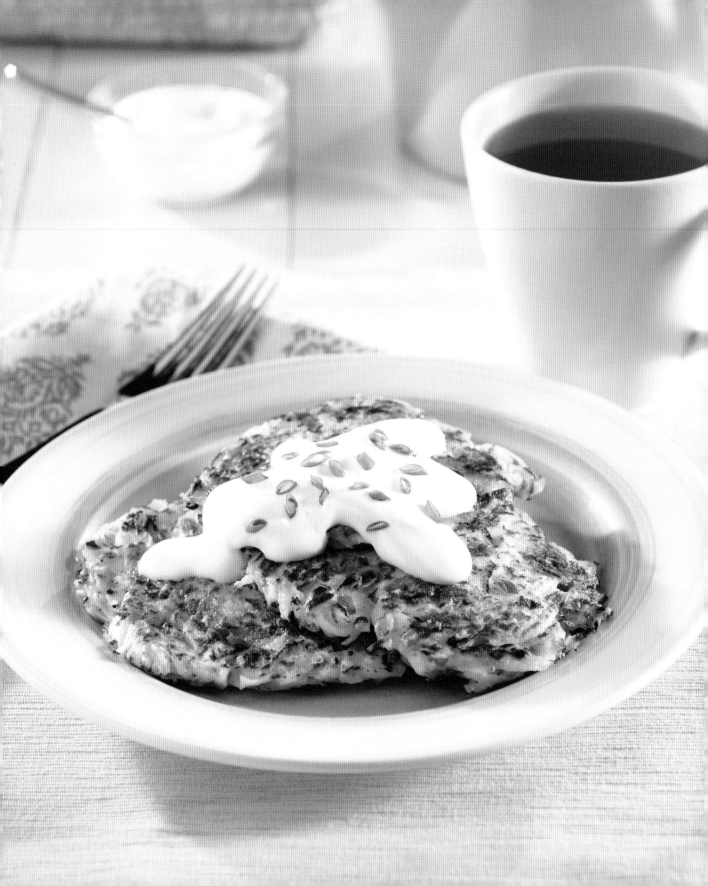

SIDE DISHES

MACARONI AND CHEESE WITH MIXED VEGETABLES

1¼ cups fat-free (skim) milk, divided
2 tablespoons all-purpose flour
½ cup (2 ounces) shredded reduced-fat sharp Cheddar cheese
½ cup (2 ounces) shredded Parmesan cheese
1½ cups frozen mixed vegetables, cooked according to package directions
1⅓ cups cooked whole wheat elbow macaroni, rotini or penne pasta
¼ teaspoon salt (optional)
⅛ teaspoon black pepper

1. Preheat oven to 325°F. Spray 1½-quart baking dish with nonstick cooking spray.

2. Stir ¼ cup milk and flour in medium saucepan until smooth and well blended. Stir in remaining 1 cup milk until well blended. Cook over medium heat until thickened, stirring constantly.

3. Combine cheeses in medium bowl. Stir half of cheese mixture into saucepan. Add vegetables, macaroni, salt, if desired, and pepper. Spoon mixture into prepared baking dish. Sprinkle evenly with remaining half of cheese mixture.

4. Bake 20 minutes or until cheese is melted and macaroni is heated through. Let stand 5 minutes before serving.
Makes 4 servings

Nutrients per Serving: *¾ cup*
Calories: 240, **Calories from Fat:** 24%, **Total Fat:** 6g,
Saturated Fat: 4g, **Cholesterol:** 20mg, **Sodium:** 330mg,
Carbohydrate: 32g, **Fiber:** 5g, **Protein:** 15g

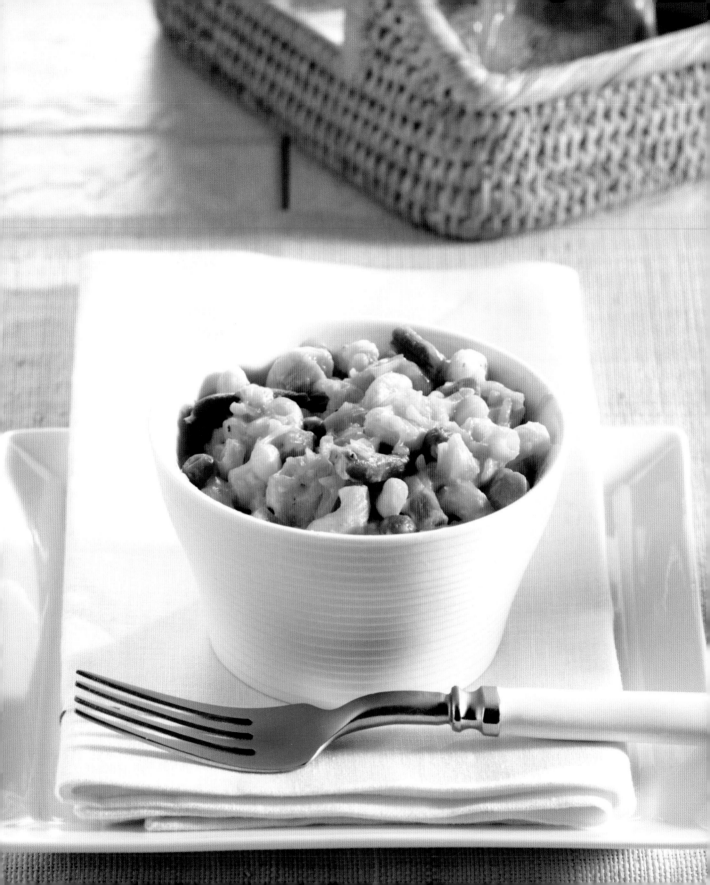

QUICK MASHED POTATOES WITH CAULIFLOWER

16 ounces russet potatoes, peeled and cut into 2-inch chunks
1 small cauliflower, trimmed into florets (about 4 to 5 cups)
¼ cup water
2 tablespoons vegetable oil spread
2 cloves garlic, minced
½ teaspoon salt
¼ teaspoon black pepper
2 tablespoons chopped chives

1. Place potatoes in medium saucepan; cover with water. Cover; bring to a boil. Reduce heat; simmer 15 minutes or until tender. Drain.

2. Meanwhile, place cauliflower and ¼ cup water in large microwavable dish. Cover; microwave on HIGH 5 minutes or until just tender. Drain.

3. Combine potatoes and cauliflower in large bowl. Mash with potato masher. Stir in vegetable oil spread, garlic, salt and pepper until spread is melted and mixture is smooth. Sprinkle with chives.

Makes 4 servings

Nutrients per Serving: ¾ *cup*
Calories: 168, **Calories from Fat:** 27%, **Total Fat:** 5g,
Saturated Fat: 1g, **Cholesterol:** 0mg, **Sodium:** 364mg,
Carbohydrate: 28g, **Fiber:** 4g, **Protein:** 4g

Note: Adding mashed cauliflower to mashed potatoes cuts down on calories and carbohydrates.

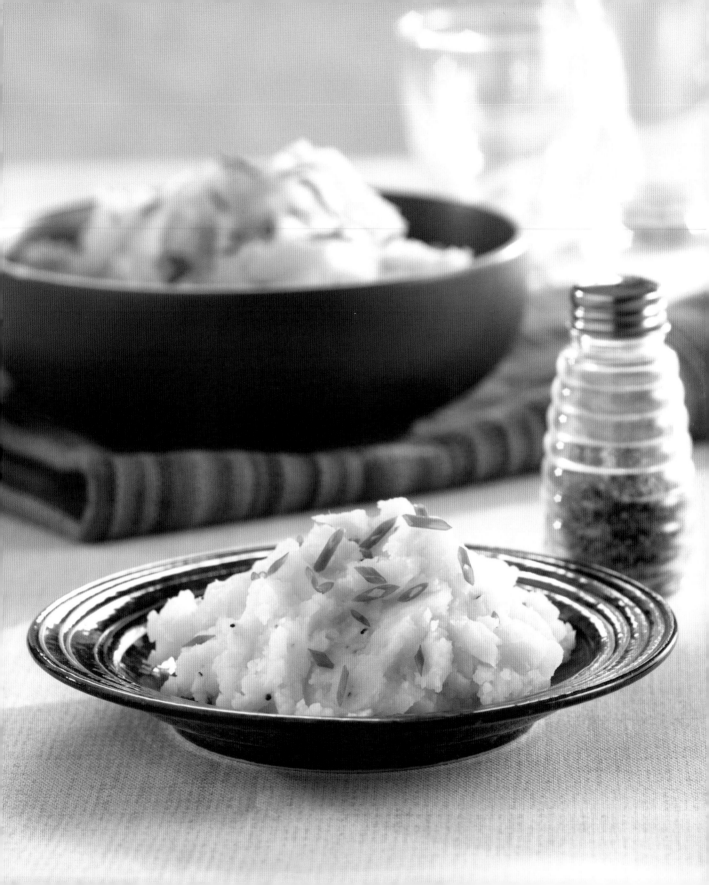

DESSERTS

STRAWBERRY-BANANA GRANITÉ

2 frozen peeled and sliced bananas (about 2 cups)

2 cups unsweetened frozen strawberries

¼ cup no-sugar-added strawberry pourable fruit*

   Whole fresh strawberries (optional)

   Fresh mint leaves (optional)

*3 tablespoons no-sugar-added strawberry fruit spread combined with 1 tablespoon warm water can be substituted.

1. Combine banana slices and frozen strawberries in food processor or blender. Let stand 10 minutes to soften fruit.

3. Add pourable fruit to strawberries and bananas in food processor; process until smooth, scraping sides of container frequently. Divide mixture among five dessert dishes. Garnish with fresh strawberries and mint leaves. Serve immediately.

Makes 5 servings

Nutrients per Serving: *⅔ cup*
Calories: 87, **Calories from Fat:** 3%, **Total Fat:** <1g,
Saturated Fat: <1g, **Cholesterol:** 0mg, **Sodium:** 2mg,
Carbohydrate: 22g, **Fiber:** 2g, **Protein:** 1g

Note: Granité can be transferred to airtight container and frozen up to 1 month. Let stand at room temperature 10 minutes to soften slightly before serving.

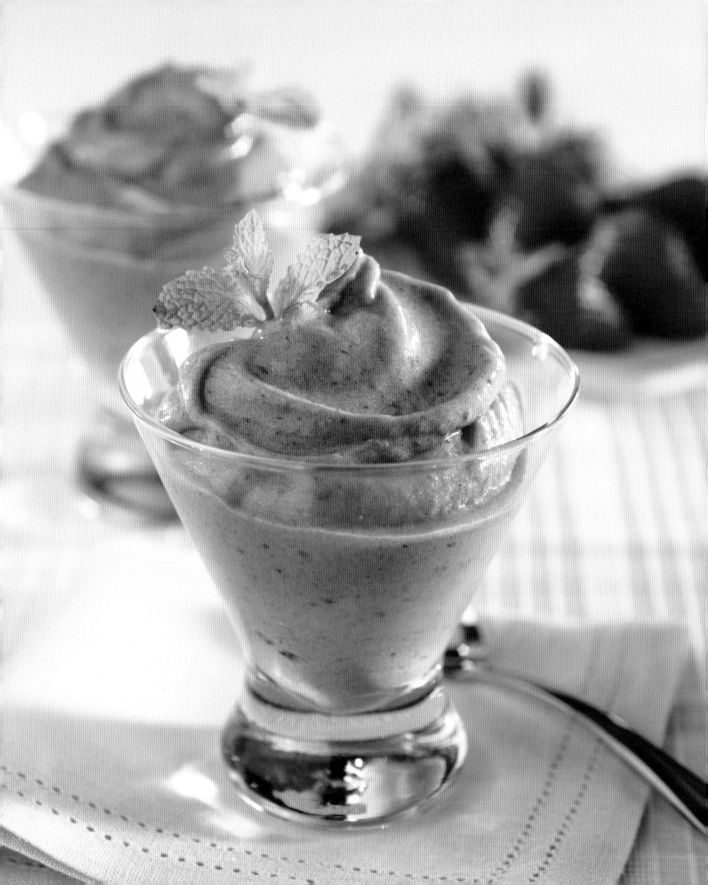

APPLE GALETTE

¾ cup all-purpose flour

¼ cup whole wheat flour

1 teaspoon baking powder

⅛ teaspoon salt

¼ cup (½ stick) cold margarine

3 tablespoons plus 1 teaspoon cold fat-free (skim) milk, divided

3 cups thinly sliced peeled baking apples

2 tablespoons sugar

1 teaspoon ground cinnamon

1. Preheat oven to 375°F.

2. Combine flours, baking powder and salt in medium bowl; mix well. Cut in margarine with pastry blender or two knives until mixture resembles coarse crumbs. Add 3 tablespoons milk, 1 tablespoon at a time, mixing with fork until dough is moistened. (Dough will be crumbly.)

3. Turn dough out on lightly floured surface; knead 6 to 8 times or just until dough clings together. Shape into ball; roll into 12-inch circle on heavy-duty foil. Transfer dough with foil to large baking sheet.

4. Combine apples, sugar and cinnamon in medium bowl; toss to coat evenly. Mound apple mixture in center of dough, leaving 2-inch border. Fold border up over filling. Brush top and side of crust with remaining 1 teaspoon milk. Cover edge of crust with foil.

5. Bake 15 minutes; remove foil. Bake 25 minutes or until crust is golden and apples are tender. Cool on baking sheet 10 minutes. Remove to wire rack; cool 20 minutes. Serve warm.

Makes 6 servings

Nutrients per Serving: *⅙ of total recipe*
Calories: 190, **Calories from Fat:** 38%, **Total Fat:** 8g,
Saturated Fat: 2g, **Cholesterol:** 0mg, **Sodium:** 210mg,
Carbohydrate: 28g, **Fiber:** 2g, **Protein:** 3g

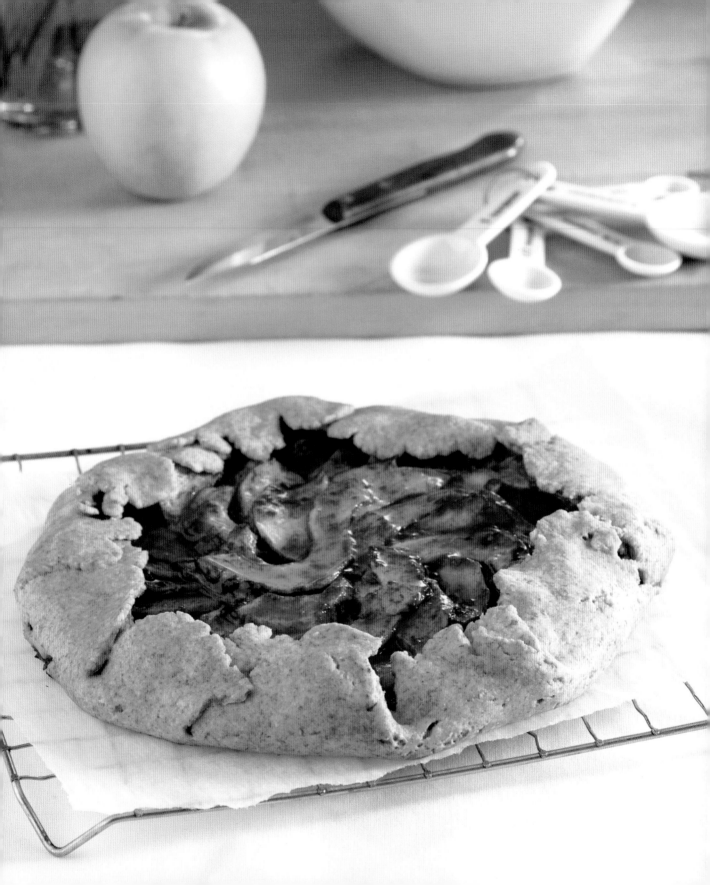

CHEWY MOCHA BROWNIE COOKIES

   1 cup all-purpose flour
¼ teaspoon baking soda
¼ cup (½ stick) margarine
⅔ cup granulated sugar
⅓ cup unsweetened cocoa powder
¼ cup packed brown sugar
1½ teaspoons instant coffee granules
¼ cup low-fat buttermilk
   1 teaspoon vanilla
   2 tablespoons powdered sugar

1. Combine flour and baking soda in small bowl; mix well. Melt margarine in medium saucepan; remove from heat. Stir in granulated sugar, cocoa, brown sugar and coffee granules until well blended. Stir in buttermilk and vanilla. Stir in flour mixture just until combined. Transfer to medium bowl. Cover and refrigerate 1 hour. (Dough will be stiff.)

2. Preheat oven to 350°F. Spray cookie sheets with nonstick cooking spray or line with parchment paper. Drop dough by rounded teaspoonfuls onto prepared cookie sheets.

3. Bake 10 to 11 minutes or until edges are firm. Cool on cookie sheets 2 minutes. Remove to wire racks; cool completely. Sprinkle with powdered sugar just before serving.

Makes about 2 dozen cookies

Nutrients per Serving: *2 cookies*
Calories: 142, **Calories from Fat:** 25%, **Total Fat:** 4g,
Saturated Fat: 1g, **Cholesterol:** 0mg, **Sodium:** 69mg,
Carbohydrate: 26g, **Fiber:** 1g, **Protein:** 2g

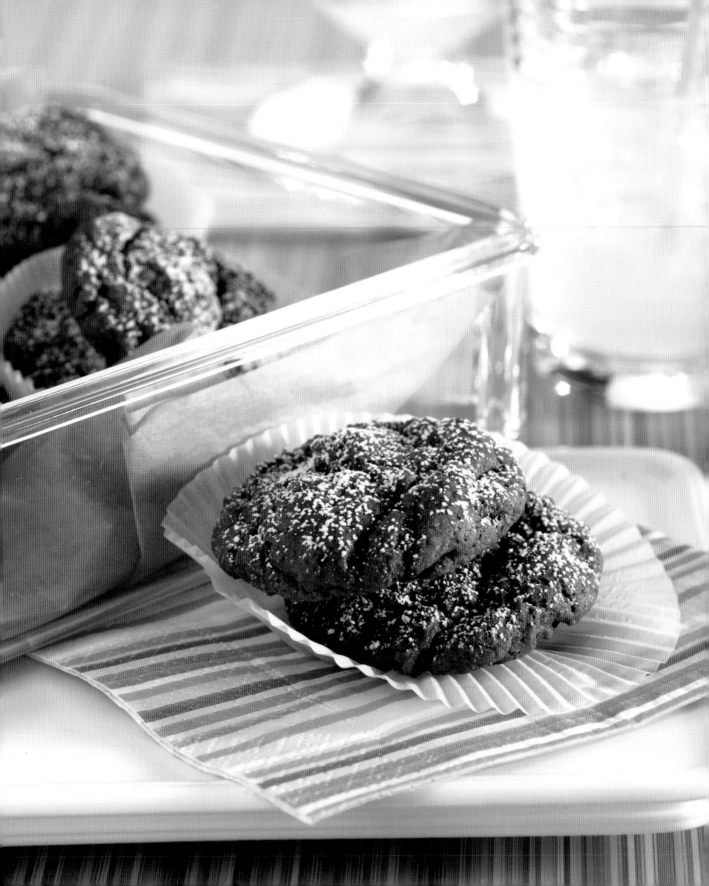

BLUEBERRY CUSTARD SUPREME

½ cup fresh blueberries
2 tablespoons all-purpose flour
1½ tablespoons granulated sugar
¼ teaspoon ground cardamom
⅛ teaspoon salt
¾ cup reduced-fat (2%) milk
¼ cup cholesterol-free egg substitute
1 teaspoon grated lemon peel
½ teaspoon vanilla
1 teaspoon powdered sugar

1. Preheat oven to 350°F. Spray 1-quart casserole or soufflé dish with nonstick cooking spray. Spread blueberries in prepared casserole.

2. Combine flour, granulated sugar, cardamom and salt in small bowl; mix well. Stir in milk, egg substitute, lemon peel and vanilla until smooth and well blended. Pour over blueberries.

3. Bake 30 minutes or until puffed, lightly browned and center is set. Cool on wire rack 10 minutes.

4. Divide custard between two dessert dishes; serve warm or at room temperature. Sprinkle with powdered sugar just before serving. *Makes 2 servings*

Nutrients per Serving: *½ of total recipe*
Calories: 155, **Calories from Fat:** 11%, **Total Fat:** 2g,
Saturated Fat: 1g, **Cholesterol:** 7mg, **Sodium:** 249mg,
Carbohydrate: 27g, **Fiber:** 1g, **Protein:** 7g

Blackberry Custard Supreme: Substitute fresh blackberries for the blueberries.

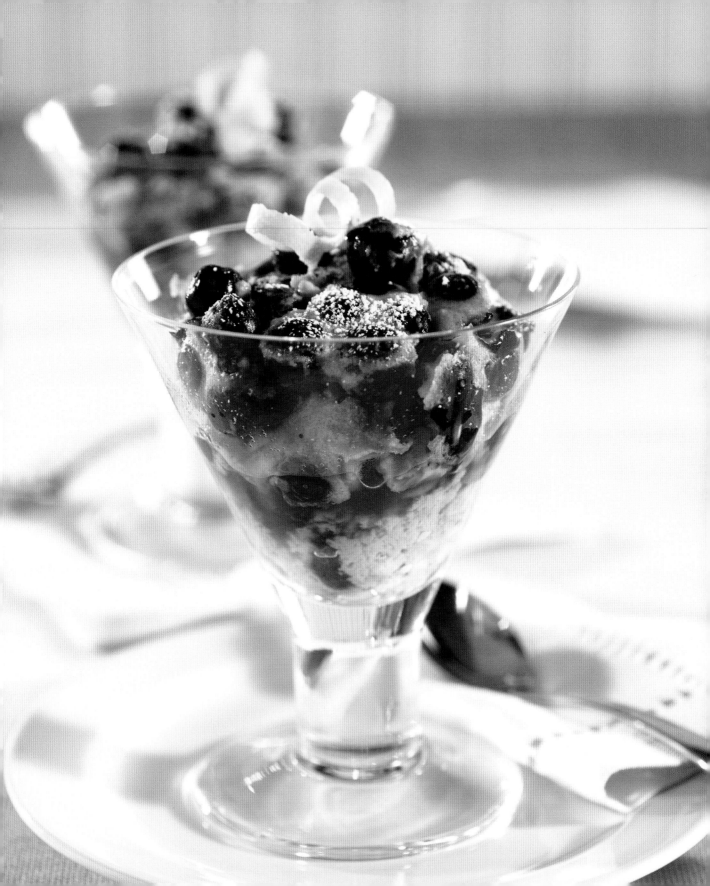

HOMEMADE COCONUT MERINGUES

   3 egg whites
   ¼ teaspoon cream of tartar
   ⅛ teaspoon salt
   ¾ cup sugar
   2¼ cups flaked coconut, toasted*
   1 teaspoon vanilla

To toast coconut, spread evenly on baking sheet. Bake in preheated 350°F oven 5 to 7 minutes or until light golden brown, stirring occasionally. Cool before using.

1. Preheat oven to 300°F. Line cookie sheets with parchment paper or foil.

2. Beat egg whites, cream of tartar and salt in large bowl with electric mixer at high speed until soft peaks form. Beat in sugar, 1 tablespoon at a time, until egg whites are stiff and shiny. Fold in coconut and vanilla. Drop dough by tablespoonfuls 2 inches apart onto prepared cookie sheets; flatten slightly.

3. Bake 18 to 22 minutes or until golden brown. Cool on cookie sheets 1 minute. Remove to wire racks; cool completely. Store in airtight container.

Makes about 2 dozen meringues

Nutrients per Serving: *3 meringues*
Calories: 161, **Calories from Fat:** 41%, **Total Fat:** 8g,
Saturated Fat: 7g, **Cholesterol:** 0mg, **Sodium:** 62mg,
Carbohydrate: 23g, **Fiber:** 2g, **Protein:** 2g

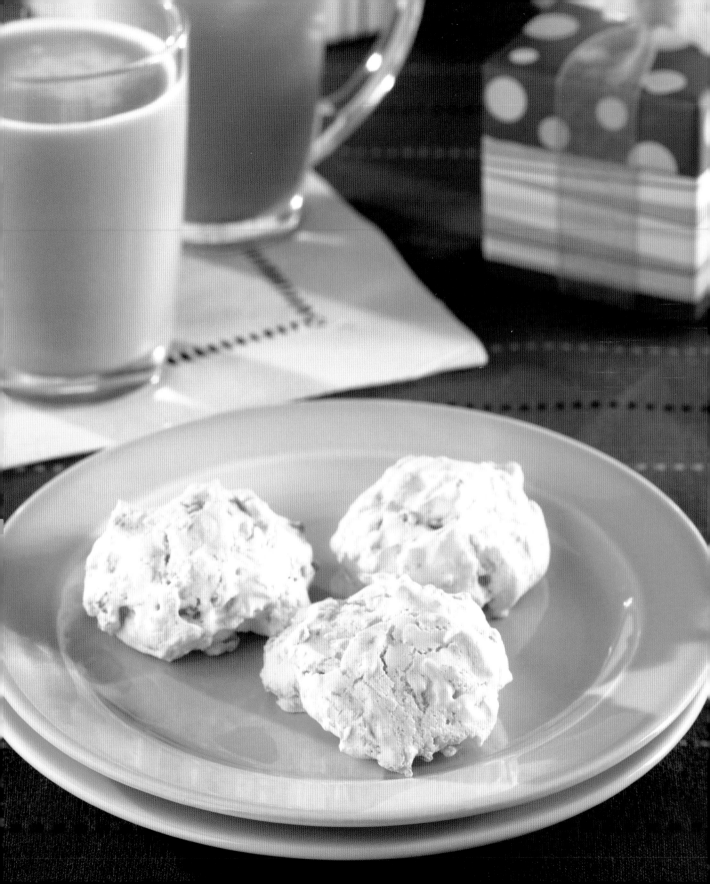

CHOCOLATE-PEANUT BUTTER CUPCAKES

1¾ cups all-purpose flour

1½ teaspoons baking powder

¼ teaspoon salt

⅓ cup (⅔ stick) butter, softened

⅓ cup creamy or chunky reduced-fat peanut butter

½ cup granulated sugar

¼ cup packed brown sugar

2 eggs

1 teaspoon vanilla

1¼ cups milk

Chocolate-Peanut Butter Frosting (page 200)

1. Preheat oven to 350°F. Line 18 standard (2½-inch) muffin cups with paper or foil baking cups.

2. Combine flour, baking powder and salt in medium bowl; mix well. Beat butter and peanut butter in large bowl with electric mixer at medium speed until smooth. Add granulated sugar and brown sugar; beat until well blended. Add eggs and vanilla; beat until well blended. Alternately add flour mixture and milk, beating well after each addition. Spoon evenly into prepared muffin cups.

3. Bake 25 minutes or until toothpick inserted into centers comes out clean. Cool in pans 10 minutes. Remove to wire racks; cool completely.

4. Prepare Chocolate-Peanut Butter Frosting. Frost cupcakes. *Makes 18 cupcakes*

Nutrients per Serving: *1 cupcake*
Calories: 201, **Calories from Fat:** 30%, **Total Fat:** 7g,
Saturated Fat: 2g, **Cholesterol:** 18mg, **Sodium:** 134mg,
Carbohydrate: 32g, **Fiber:** 1g, **Protein:** 4g

continued on page 200

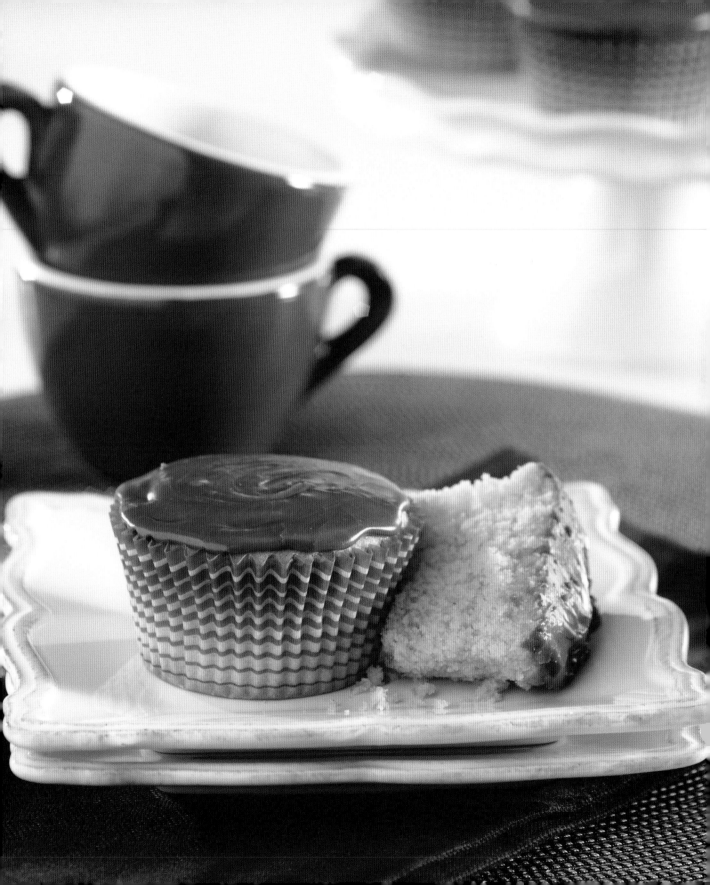

Chocolate-Peanut Butter Cupcakes, continued

CHOCOLATE-PEANUT BUTTER FROSTING

4 cups powdered sugar
⅓ cup unsweetened cocoa powder
4 to 6 tablespoons milk, divided
3 tablespoons creamy peanut butter

Beat powdered sugar, cocoa, 4 tablespoons milk and peanut butter in large bowl with electric mixer at low speed until smooth. Beat in additional milk, 1 tablespoon at a time, until desired spreading consistency is reached. *Makes about 2½ cups*

FRUIT KABOBS WITH RASPBERRY YOGURT DIP

½ cup plain nonfat yogurt
¼ cup no-sugar-added raspberry fruit spread
1 pint fresh strawberries
2 cups cubed honeydew melon (1-inch cubes)
2 cups cubed cantaloupe (1-inch cubes)
1 can (8 ounces) pineapple chunks in juice, drained

Stir yogurt and fruit spread in small bowl until well blended. Alternately thread fruit onto six 12-inch skewers. Serve with yogurt dip. *Makes 6 servings*

Nutrients per Serving: *1 kabob with about 2 tablespoons dip*
Calories: 108, **Calories from Fat:** 3%, **Total Fat:** <1g,
Saturated Fat: <1g, **Cholesterol:** <1mg, **Sodium:** 52mg,
Carbohydrate: 25g, **Fiber:** 2g, **Protein:** 2g

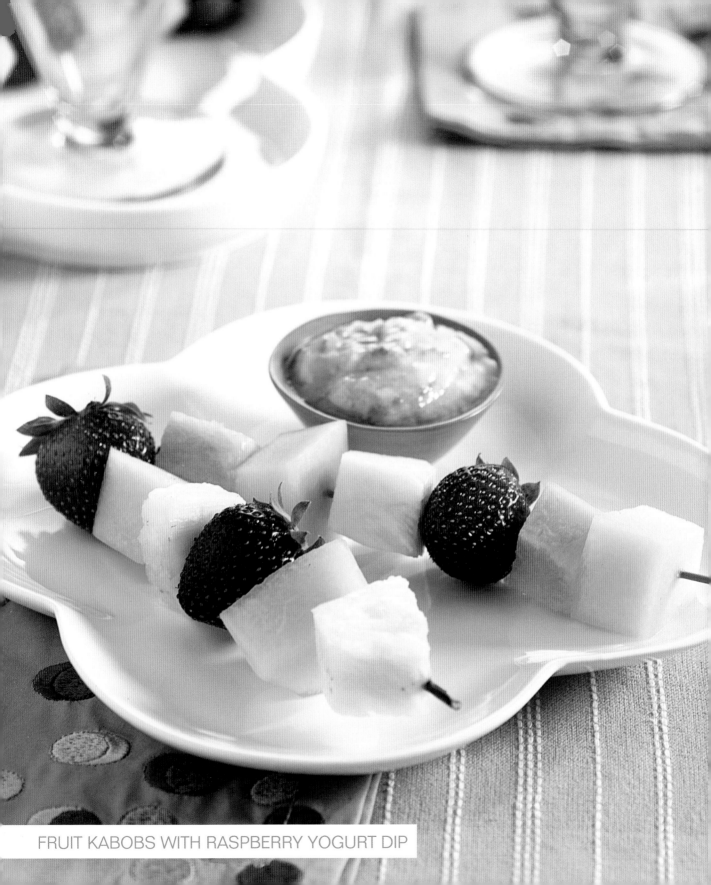

FRUIT KABOBS WITH RASPBERRY YOGURT DIP

PINEAPPLE-RAISIN SQUARES

2 eggs

1 cup thawed frozen unsweetened pineapple juice concentrate

¼ cup butter, melted

1 teaspoon vanilla

1⅓ cups all-purpose flour

⅔ cup old-fashioned oats

1 teaspoon baking soda

1 teaspoon ground cinnamon

½ teaspoon ground ginger

¼ teaspoon salt

⅛ teaspoon ground nutmeg

1 can (8 ounces) crushed pineapple in unsweetened juice, well drained

¾ cup chopped pecans, lightly toasted*

½ cup golden raisins

To toast pecans, spread in a single layer on ungreased baking sheet. Bake in preheated 350°F oven 6 to 8 minutes or until fragrant, stirring occasionally.

1. Preheat oven to 350°F. Spray 12×8-inch baking dish with nonstick cooking spray.

2. Beat eggs in large bowl. Stir in pineapple juice concentrate, butter and vanilla until well blended. Add flour, oats, baking soda, cinnamon, ginger, salt and nutmeg; mix well. Stir in crushed pineapple, pecans and raisins. Spoon batter into prepared dish.

3. Bake 18 to 20 minutes or until set. Cool completely on wire rack; cut into squares. Store in airtight container. *Makes 16 squares*

Nutrients per Serving: *1 square*
Calories: 181, **Calories from Fat:** 38%, **Total Fat:** 8g,
Saturated Fat: 2g, **Cholesterol:** 35mg, **Sodium:** 156mg,
Carbohydrate: 26g, **Fiber:** 2g, **Protein:** 3g

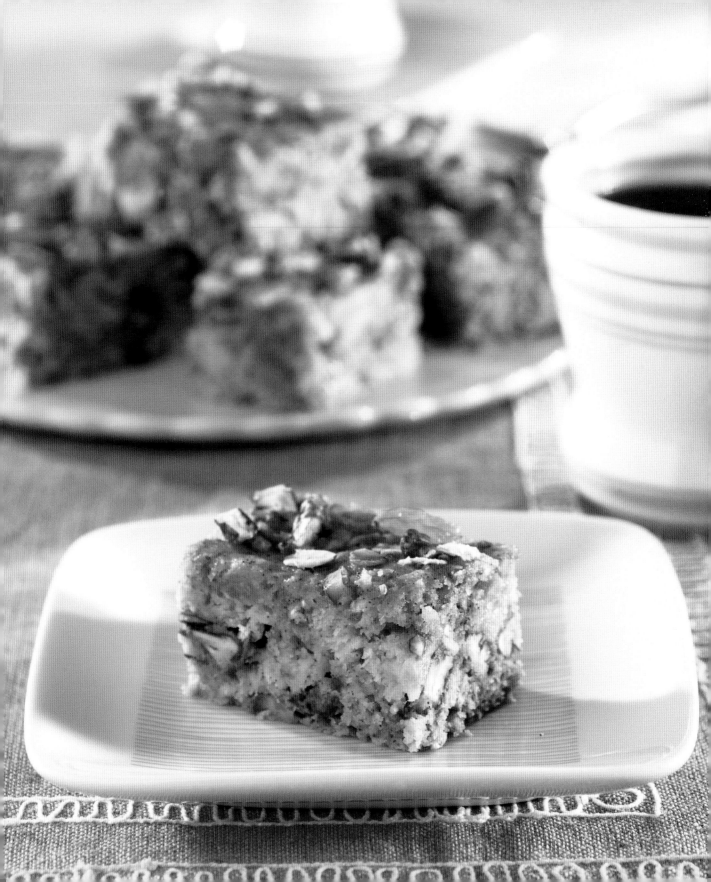

CINNAMON DESSERT TACOS WITH FRUIT SALSA

1 cup sliced fresh strawberries

1 cup cubed fresh pineapple

1 cup cubed peeled kiwi

½ teaspoon minced jalapeño pepper* (optional)

3 tablespoons sugar

1 tablespoon ground cinnamon

6 (8-inch) flour tortillas

Nonstick cooking spray

*Jalapeño peppers can sting and irritate the skin, so wear rubber gloves when handling peppers and do not touch your eyes.

1. Combine strawberries, pineapple, kiwi and jalapeño in large bowl; set aside. Combine sugar and cinnamon in small bowl; set aside.

2. Working with one tortilla at a time, spray lightly on both sides with cooking spray; place in large nonstick skillet. Heat over medium heat until slightly puffed and golden brown. Remove from heat; immediately dust both sides with cinnamon-sugar mixture, letting excess cinnamon-sugar shake back into bowl. Repeat with remaining tortillas.

3. Spoon fruit mixture evenly down centers of tortillas; fold in half. Serve immediately.

Makes 6 servings

Nutrients per Serving: *1 dessert taco with about ⅙ of fruit salsa*
Calories: 183, **Calories from Fat:** 14%, **Total Fat:** 3g,
Saturated Fat: <1g, **Cholesterol:** 0mg, **Sodium:** 169mg,
Carbohydrate: 36g, **Fiber:** 4g, **Protein:** 4g

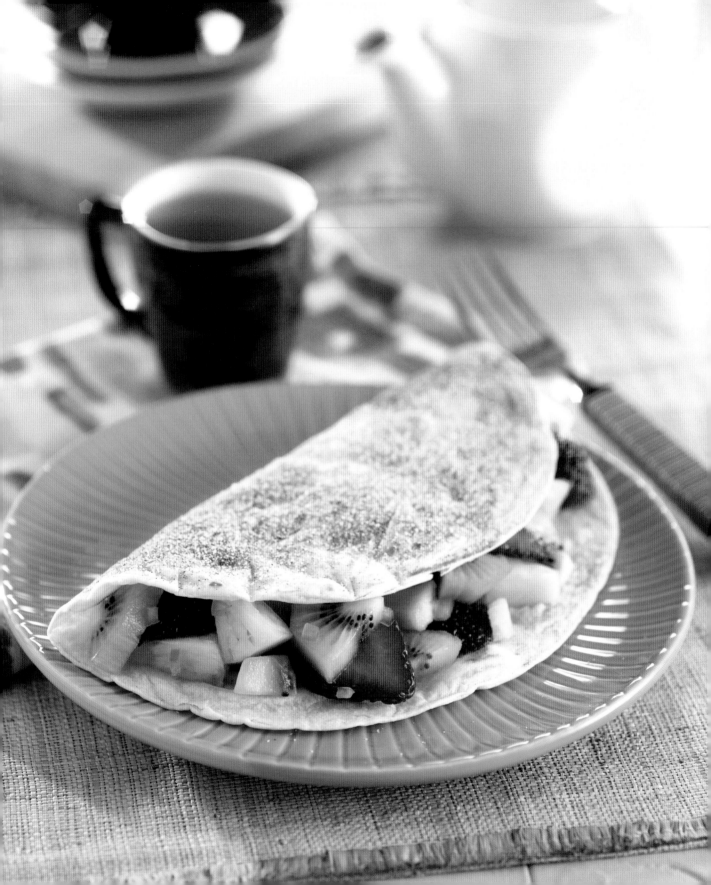

CHOCOLATE CHIP BROWNIES

¾ cup granulated sugar

½ cup butter

2 tablespoons water

2 cups semisweet chocolate chips or mini chocolate chips, divided

1½ teaspoons vanilla

1¼ cups all-purpose flour

½ teaspoon baking soda

½ teaspoon salt

2 eggs

Powdered sugar (optional)

1. Preheat oven to 350°F. Spray 9-inch square baking pan with nonstick cooking spray.

2. Combine granulated sugar, butter and water in medium microwavable bowl. Microwave on HIGH 1½ to 2 minutes or until butter is melted. Stir in 1 cup chocolate chips until chocolate is melted and mixture is smooth. Stir in vanilla; let stand 5 minutes to cool slightly.

3. Combine flour, baking soda and salt in small bowl; mix well. Add eggs to chocolate mixture, one at a time, beating well after each addition. Add flour mixture; mix well. Stir in remaining 1 cup chocolate chips. Spoon batter into prepared pan.

4. Bake 25 minutes for fudgy brownies or 30 to 35 minutes for cakelike brownies. Cool completely in pan on wire rack.

5. Cut brownies into 2¼-inch squares. Place powdered sugar in fine-mesh strainer and sprinkle over brownies, if desired. Store tightly covered at room temperature or freeze up to 3 months. *Makes 16 brownies*

Nutrients per Serving: *1 brownie*
Calories: 230, **Calories from Fat:** 51%, **Total Fat:** 13g,
Saturated Fat: 8g, **Cholesterol:** 40mg, **Sodium:** 170mg,
Carbohydrate: 30g, **Fiber:** 2g, **Protein:** 3g

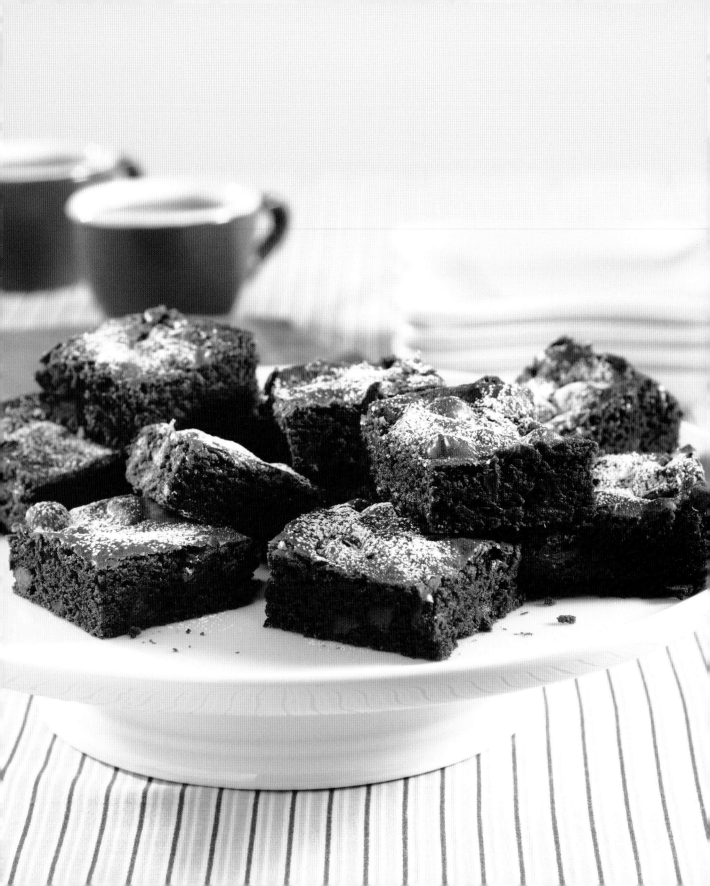

CHEWY CORNBREAD COOKIES

1 cup (2 sticks) unsalted butter, softened
⅔ cup plus 2 tablespoons sugar, divided
1 egg
1 teaspoon vanilla
½ teaspoon salt
2 cups corn flour
½ cup instant polenta

1. Beat butter and ⅔ cup sugar in large bowl with electric mixer at medium-high speed until creamy. Beat in egg, vanilla and salt until well blended. Combine corn flour and polenta in medium bowl. Gradually add to butter mixture, beating well after each addition. (Dough will be very sticky.)

2. Shape dough into two discs. Wrap in plastic wrap; refrigerate at least 2 hours.

3. Preheat oven to 350°F. Line cookie sheets with parchment paper.

4. Shape dough into 1-inch balls. Roll in remaining 2 tablespoons sugar. Place 1 inch apart on prepared cookie sheets.

5. Bake 12 to 14 minutes. Cool completely on cookie sheets.

Makes about 4 dozen cookies

Nutrients per Serving: *2 cookies*
Calories: 123, **Calories from Fat:** 61%, **Total Fat:** 8g,
Saturated Fat: 5g, **Cholesterol:** 28mg, **Sodium:** 5mg,
Carbohydrate: 11g, **Fiber:** 1g, **Protein:** 1g

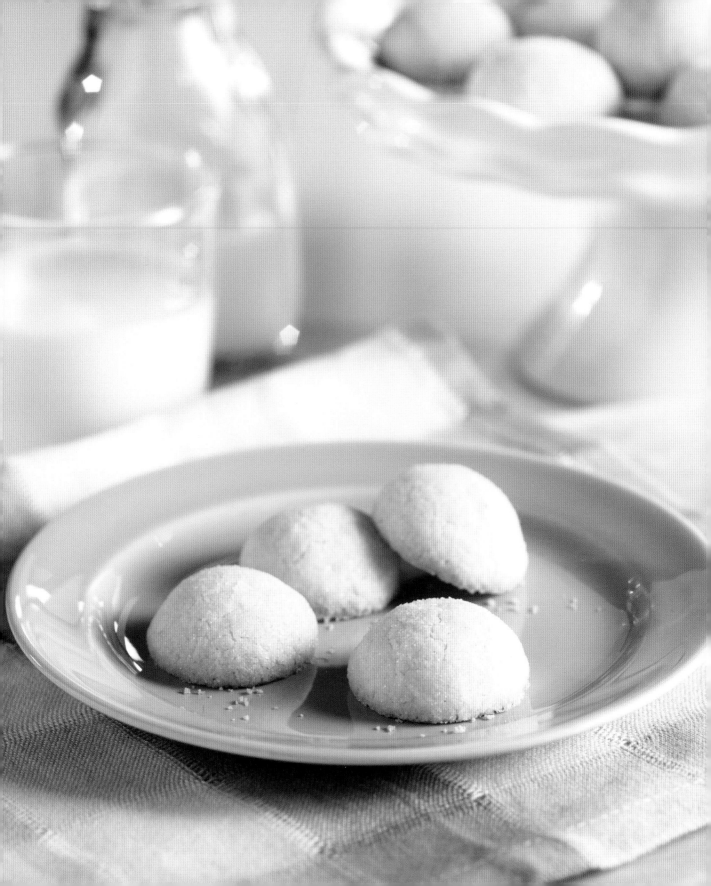

TOASTED COCONUT AND TROPICAL FRUIT PARFAITS

1 cup pineapple sherbet

1 cup diced strawberries

¾ cup diced mango or peaches

1 kiwi, peeled and diced

2 tablespoons flaked sweetened coconut*

*To toast coconut, spread in thin layer in heavy-bottomed skillet. Cook and stir over medium heat until golden, about 3 to 5 minutes. Remove from skillet immediately. Cool before using.

Scoop ¼ cup sherbet into each of four dessert dishes. Spoon strawberries, mango and kiwi evenly over sherbet. Sprinkle with coconut. Serve immediately.

Makes 4 servings

Nutrients per Serving: *1 parfait*

Calories: 110, **Calories from Fat:** 12%, **Total Fat:** 2g,
Saturated Fat: 1g, **Cholesterol:** 0mg, **Sodium:** 45mg,
Carbohydrate: 25g, **Fiber:** 3g, **Protein:** 1g

TIP   This tropical treat works well with any fruit-flavored frozen yogurt, too. You can also use any combination of your favorite fruits.

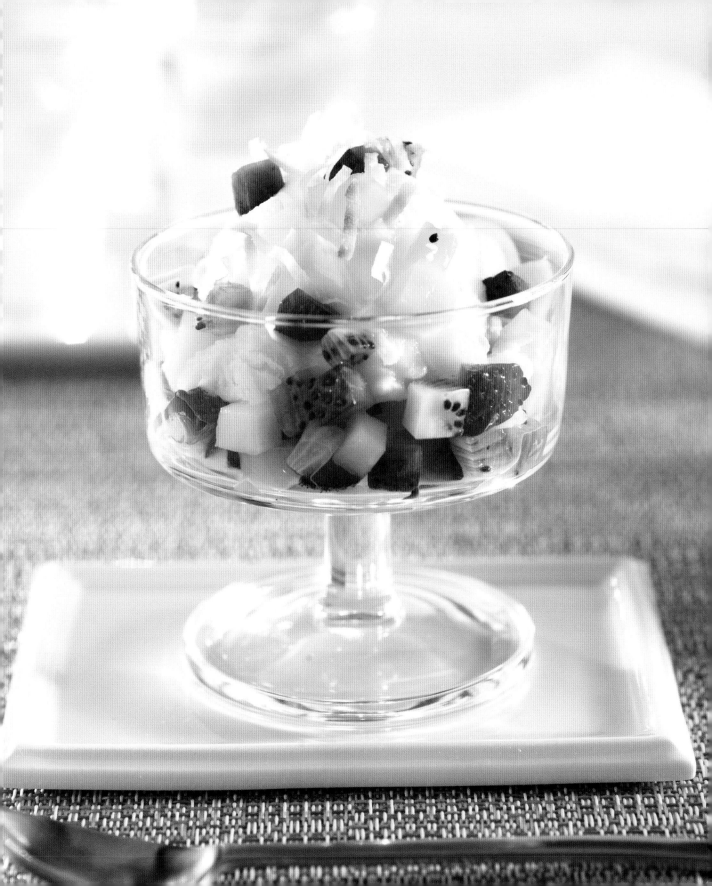

CHAI TEA GRANITA

2 cinnamon sticks

5 whole cloves

1 teaspoon cardamom seeds

3 cups water

4 black tea bags *or* ¼ cup loose black tea leaves

2 cups fat-free (skim) milk

3 tablespoons honey

½ teaspoon vanilla

1. Combine cinnamon sticks, cloves and cardamom in small cheesecloth; tie with kitchen string.

2. Bring water to a boil in medium saucepan over high heat; reduce heat. Add tea and spice bag; simmer 15 minutes.

3. Remove spices to fine-mesh strainer; strain remaining liquid from spice bag into shallow dish. Stir in milk, honey and vanilla until well combined.

4. Cover and freeze 45 minutes. Remove dish from freezer. Scrape through mixture with fork, breaking ice into fine crystals; return to freezer. Repeat at 30 minute intervals until thoroughly frozen. *Makes 4 servings*

Nutrients per Serving: ¼ *of total recipe*
Calories: 93, **Calories from Fat:** 0%, **Total Fat:** 0g,
Saturated Fat: 0g, **Cholesterol:** 2mg, **Sodium:** 58mg,
Carbohydrate: 20g, **Fiber:** 0g, **Protein:** 4g

Note: Granita, will keep, covered, up to 1 week.

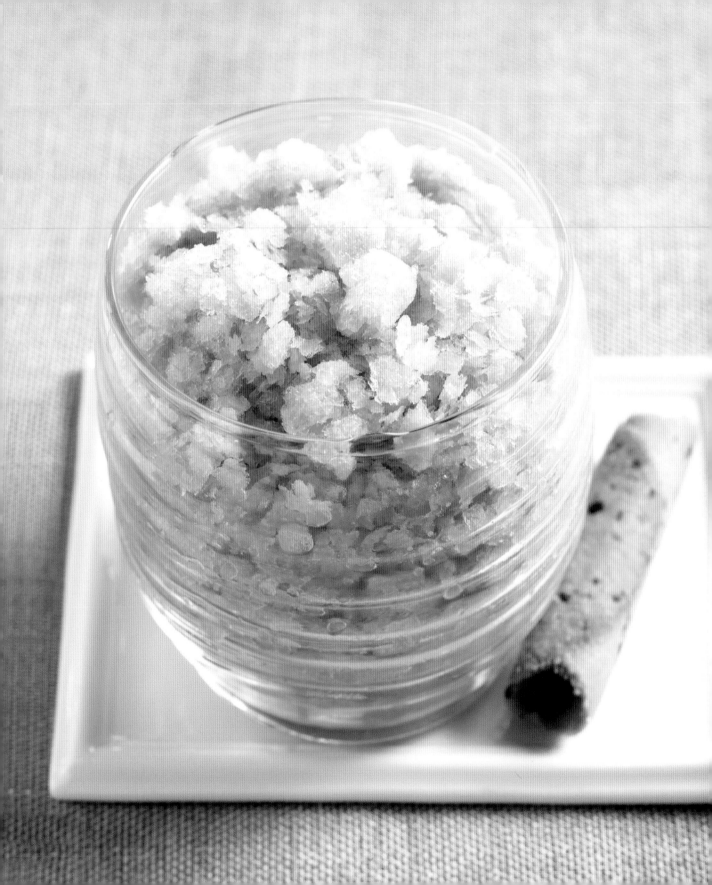

MANGO-RASPBERRY CRISP

1 mango, peeled, seeded and chopped into ½-inch pieces
1 cup fresh raspberries
½ cup old-fashioned oats
2 tablespoons packed brown sugar
½ to 1 teaspoon ground cinnamon
4 teaspoons butter
2 tablespoons chopped pecans

1. Preheat oven to 400°F. Spray four 6-ounce custard cups or ramekins with nonstick cooking spray. Divide mango and raspberries evenly among custard cups.

2. Combine oats, brown sugar and cinnamon in medium bowl; mix well. Cut in butter with pastry blender or two knives until mixture resembles coarse crumbs. Stir in pecans. Sprinkle evenly over fruit.

3. Bake 20 to 25 minutes or until fruit is tender and topping is golden brown. Let stand 15 minutes before serving. *Makes 4 servings*

Nutrients per Serving: *¼ of total recipe*
Calories: 171, **Calories from Fat:** 37%, **Total Fat:** 7g,
Saturated Fat: 3g, **Cholesterol:** 10mg, **Sodium:** 31mg,
Carbohydrate: 27g, **Fiber:** 4g, **Protein:** 2g

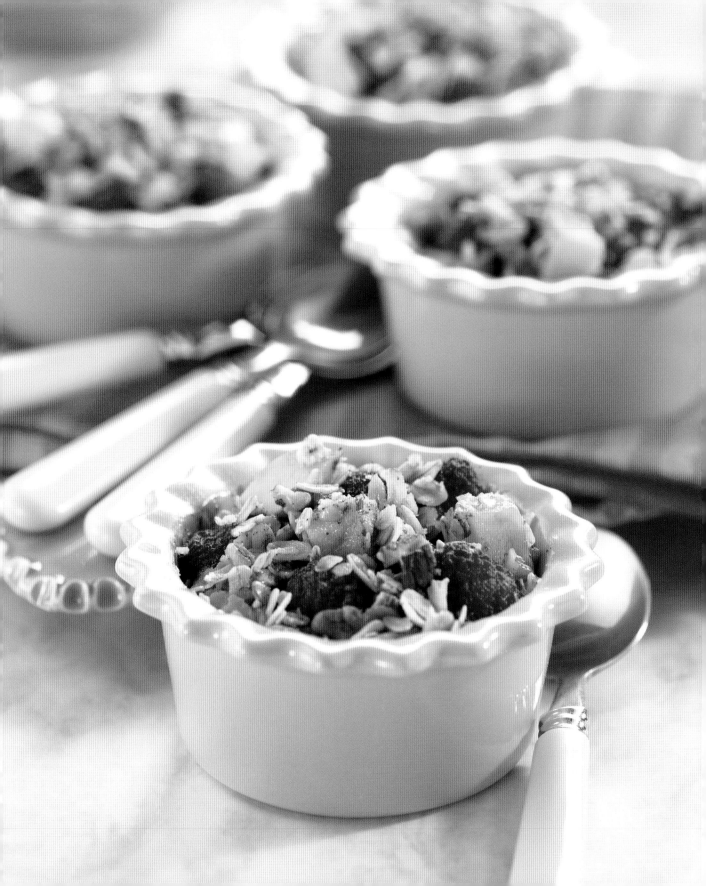

FROZEN CHOCOLATE-COVERED BANANAS

2 medium ripe bananas
4 pop sticks
½ cup granola cereal without raisins
1 bottle (7¼ ounces) quick-hardening chocolate shell dessert topping

1. Line baking sheet with waxed paper.

2. Peel bananas; cut each in half crosswise. Insert stick about 1½ inches into center of cut end of each banana. Place on prepared baking sheet. Freeze 2 hours or until firm.

3. Place granola in large resealable food storage bag; crush slightly using rolling pin or meat mallet. Transfer granola to shallow dish. Pour chocolate shell topping in separate shallow dish.

4. Place 1 frozen banana in topping; turn and spread evenly over banana with spatula. Immediately place banana in dish with granola, turning to coat evenly. Return to baking sheet. Repeat with remaining bananas.

5. Freeze 2 hours or until firm. Let stand 5 minutes before serving.   *Makes 4 servings*

Nutrients per Serving: ½ *banana*
Calories: 191, **Calories from Fat:** 19%, **Total Fat:** 4g,
Saturated Fat: 2g, **Cholesterol:** 3mg, **Sodium:** 132mg,
Carbohydrate: 38g, **Fiber:** 3g, **Protein:** 3g

TIP   For a fun twist on these treats, roll in coconut, chopped peanuts or any other desired toppings.

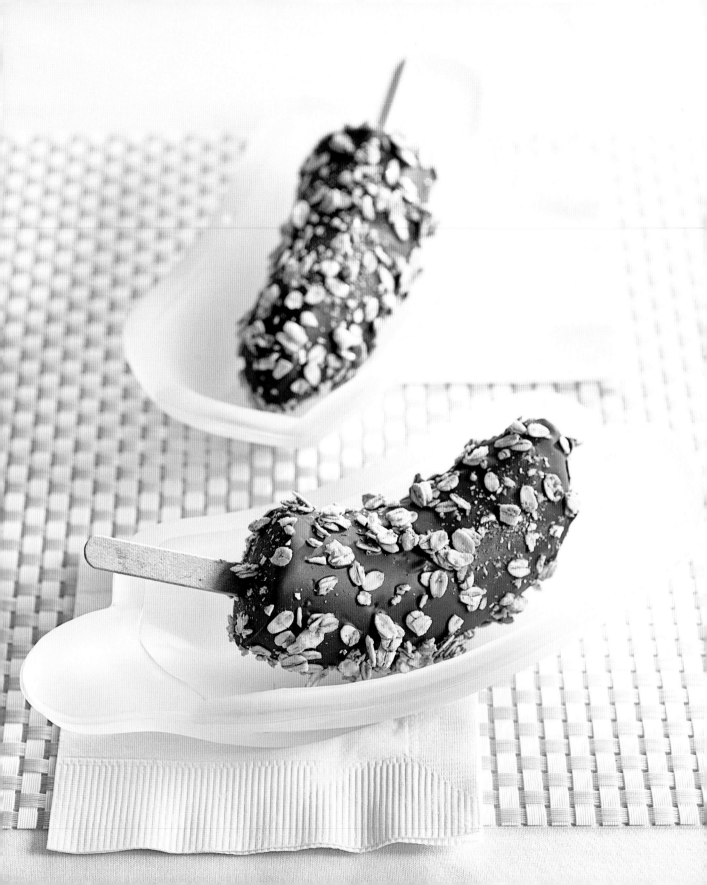

SNACKS

VEGETABLE-TOPPED HUMMUS

    1 can (about 15 ounces) chickpeas, rinsed and drained

    2 tablespoons tahini*

    2 tablespoons lemon juice

    1 clove garlic

    ¾ teaspoon salt

    1 tomato, finely chopped

    2 green onions, finely chopped

    2 tablespoons chopped fresh parsley

      Pita bread wedges or assorted crackers (optional)

*Tahini is a thick paste made of ground sesame seeds used in Middle Eastern cooking.

1. Combine chickpeas, tahini, lemon juice, garlic and salt in food processor or blender; process until smooth.

2. Combine tomato, green onions and parsley in small bowl; gently toss to combine.

3. Spoon chickpea mixture into serving bowl; top with tomato mixture. Serve with pita wedges, if desired. *Makes 8 servings*

Nutrients per Serving: *6 tablespoons*
Calories: 75, **Calories from Fat:** 36%, **Total Fat:** 3g,
Saturated Fat: 0g, **Cholesterol:** 0mg, **Sodium:** 369mg,
Carbohydrate: 9g, **Fiber:** 3g, **Protein:** 4g

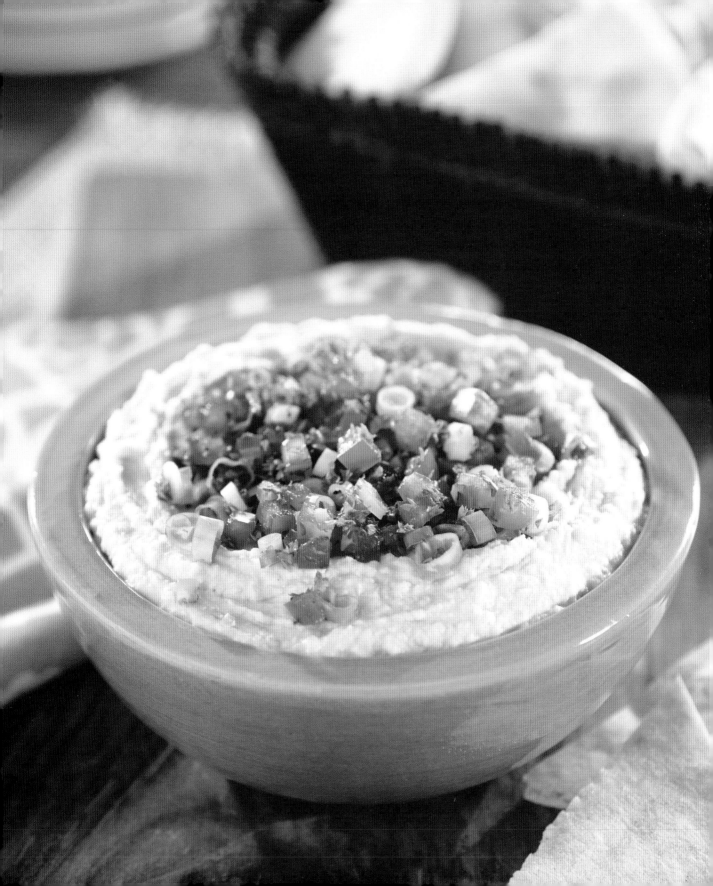

WILD WEDGES

2 (8-inch) fat-free flour tortillas
   Nonstick cooking spray
⅓ cup shredded reduced-fat Cheddar cheese
⅓ cup chopped cooked chicken or turkey
1 green onion, thinly sliced
2 tablespoons mild thick and chunky salsa

Heat large nonstick skillet over medium heat. Spray one side of 1 tortilla with cooking spray; place in skillet, sprayed side down. Top with cheese, chicken, green onion and salsa. Place remaining tortilla on top; spray with cooking spray. Cook 2 to 3 minutes per side or until golden brown and cheese is melted. To serve, cut into eight wedges.

Makes 4 servings

Nutrients per Serving: *2 wedges*
Calories: 82, **Calories from Fat:** 25%, **Total Fat:** 2g,
Saturated Fat: 1g, **Cholesterol:** 13mg, **Sodium:** 224mg,
Carbohydrate: 8g, **Fiber:** 3g, **Protein:** 7g

TIP   For a vegetarian option, omit the chicken and spread ⅓ cup canned fat-free refried beans over one of the tortillas.

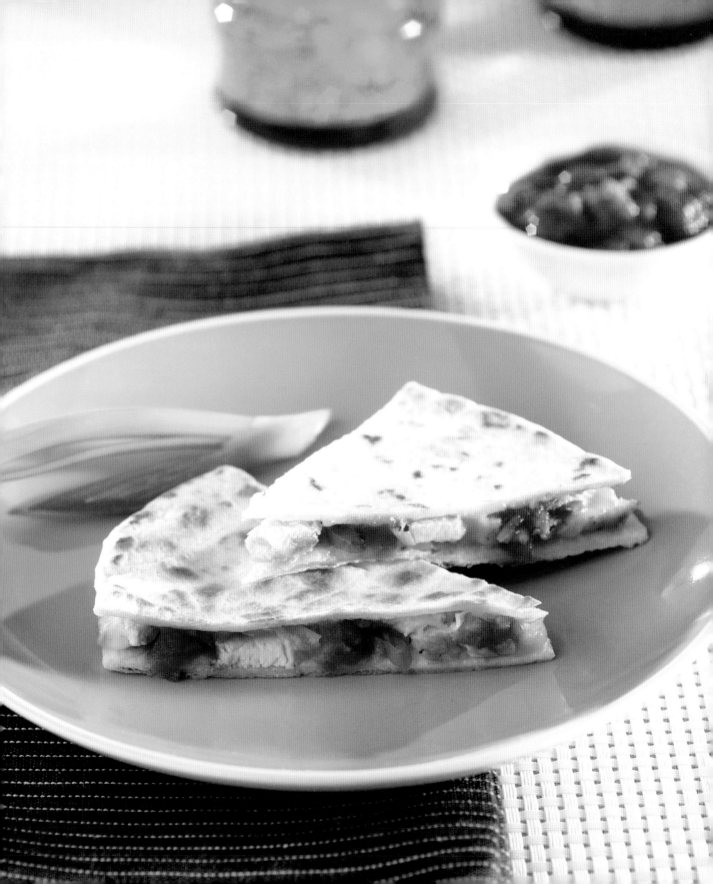

CREAMY CASHEW SPREAD

1 cup raw cashews
2 tablespoons lemon juice
1 tablespoon tahini*
½ teaspoon salt
½ teaspoon freshly ground pepper
2 teaspoons minced fresh herbs, such as basil, parsley or oregano (optional)
Tahini is a thick paste made of ground sesame seeds used in Middle Eastern cooking.

1. Rinse cashews and place in medium bowl. Cover with water by at least 2 inches. Soak 4 hours or overnight.

2. Drain cashews, reserving soaking water. Combine cashews, lemon juice, tahini, salt, pepper and 2 tablespoons soaking water in food processor; process 4 to 6 minutes or until smooth. Add additional water, 1 tablespoon at a time, until desired consistency is reached, if necessary.

3. Refrigerate until ready to serve. Stir in herbs just before serving.

Makes ½ cup (about 6 servings)

Nutrients per Serving: *1⅓ tablespoons*
Calories: 136, **Calories from Fat:** 66%, **Total Fat:** 11g,
Saturated Fat: 2g, **Cholesterol:** 0mg, **Sodium:** 197mg,
Carbohydrate: 8g, **Fiber:** 1g, **Protein:** 4g

Serving Suggestion: Use as a spread or dip with vegetables or crackers. It even works well on toast.

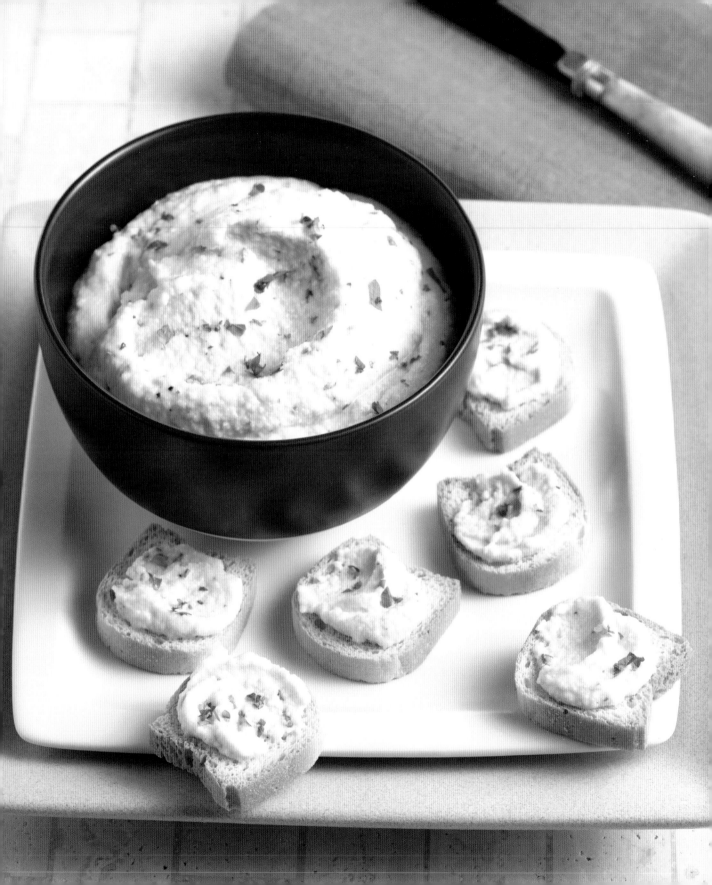

STRAWBERRY OAT MINI MUFFINS

    1 cup all-purpose flour
    ¾ cup uncooked oat bran cereal
  2½ teaspoons baking powder
    ½ teaspoon baking soda
    ⅛ teaspoon salt
    ¾ cup buttermilk
    ⅓ cup frozen apple juice concentrate, thawed
    ⅓ cup unsweetened applesauce
    ½ teaspoon vanilla
    ¾ cup diced strawberries
    ¼ cup chopped pecans

1. Preheat oven to 400°F. Spray 24 mini (1¾-inch) muffin cups with nonstick cooking spray.

2. Combine flour, cereal, baking powder, baking soda and salt in medium bowl; mix well. Whisk buttermilk, apple juice concentrate, applesauce and vanilla in small bowl until well blended. Stir buttermilk mixture into flour mixture just until moistened. Fold in strawberries and pecans. *Do not overmix.* Spoon evenly into prepared muffin cups.

3. Bake 17 to 18 minutes or until lightly browned and toothpick inserted into centers comes out clean. Cool in pans on wire racks 5 minutes. Remove to wire racks; serve warm or cool completely.

Makes 24 mini muffins

Nutrients per Serving: *3 mini muffins*
Calories: 135, **Calories from Fat:** 21%, **Total Fat:** 3g,
Saturated Fat: <1g, **Cholesterol:** 1mg, **Sodium:** 310mg,
Carbohydrate: 23g, **Fiber:** 2g, **Protein:** 4g

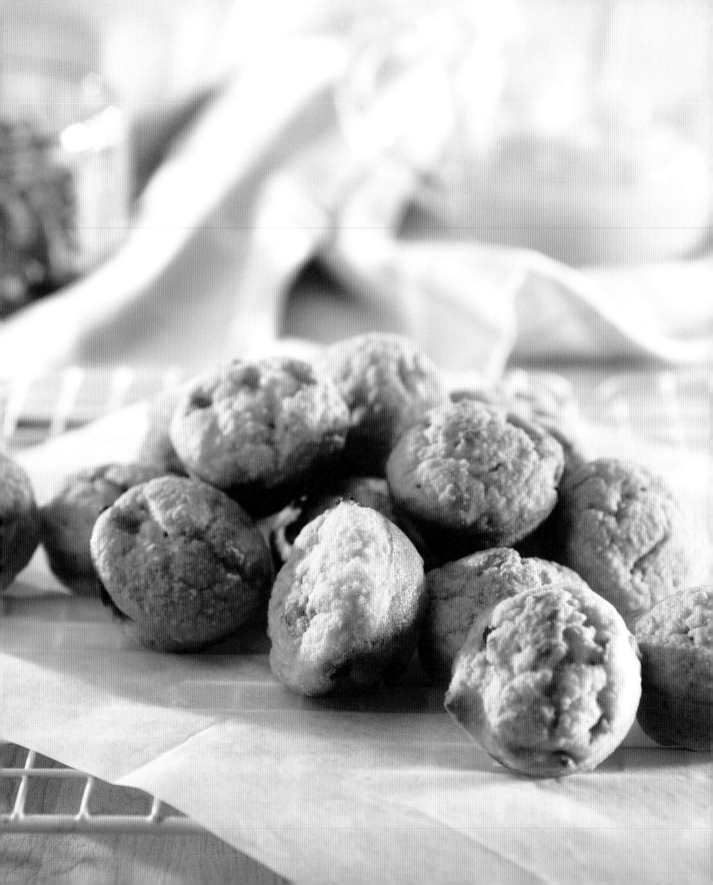

TORTELLINI TEASERS

    Zesty Tomato Sauce (recipe follows)
  ½ (9-ounce) package refrigerated cheese tortellini
  1 large red or green bell pepper, cut into 1-inch pieces
  2 medium carrots, cut into ½-inch pieces
  1 medium zucchini, cut into ½-inch pieces
 12 medium mushrooms
 12 cherry tomatoes

1. Prepare Zesty Tomato Sauce; keep warm.

2. Cook tortellini according to package directions. Drain.

3. Alternately thread tortellini and vegetable pieces on wooden skewers. Serve as dippers with Zesty Tomato Sauce. *Makes 6 servings*

Nutrients per Serving: *1 kabob with about ¼ cup*
Zesty Tomato Sauce
Calories: 130, **Calories from Fat:** 15%, **Total Fat:** 2g,
Saturated Fat: 1g, **Cholesterol:** 12mg, **Sodium:** 306mg,
Carbohydrate: 23g, **Fiber:** 5g, **Protein:** 7g

ZESTY TOMATO SAUCE

  1 can (15 ounces) tomato purée
  2 tablespoons finely chopped onion
  2 tablespoons chopped fresh parsley
  1 teaspoon dried oregano
 ¼ teaspoon dried thyme
 ¼ teaspoon salt
 ⅛ teaspoon black pepper

Combine tomato purée, onion, parsley, oregano and thyme in small saucepan. Heat thoroughly, stirring occasionally. Stir in salt and pepper. *Makes about 1⅔ cups*

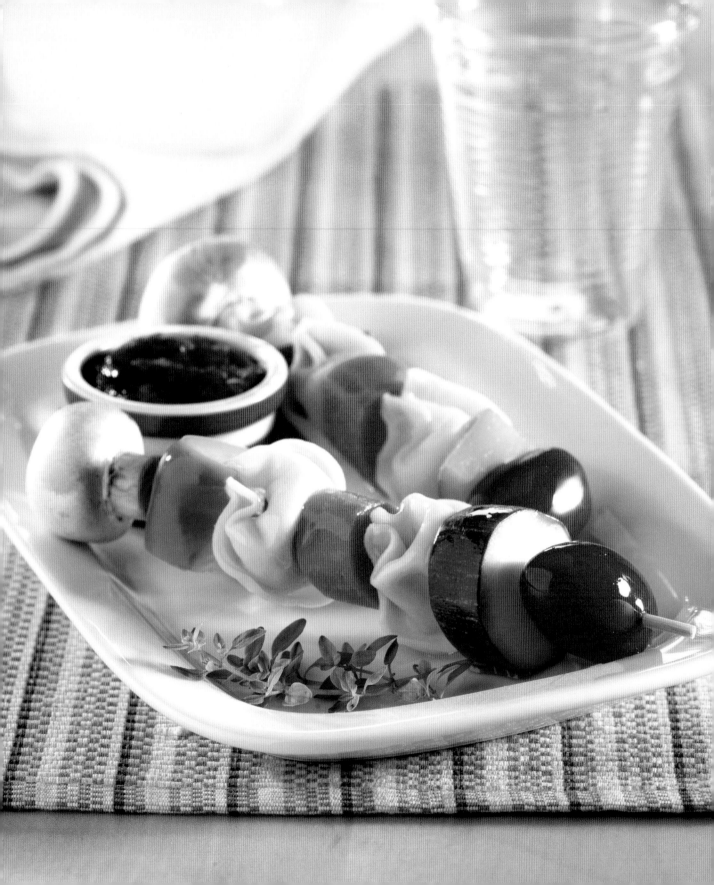

CRISPY SWEET SNACK BARS

3 tablespoons creamy peanut butter

2 tablespoons molasses

2 egg whites

2 tablespoons ground flax seeds

4 cups crisp rice cereal

½ cup sliced almonds

1 ounce bittersweet chocolate, melted

1. Preheat oven to 350°F. Spray 9-inch square baking pan with nonstick cooking spray. Place peanut butter in small microwavable bowl; microwave on LOW (30%) 30 seconds or until peanut butter is melted. Stir in molasses; set aside to cool completely.

2. Place egg whites and flax seeds in blender or food processor; blend until foamy. Pour into large bowl. Add peanut butter mixture; stir until smooth. Stir in cereal and almonds until cereal is evenly coated. Press cereal mixture into prepared pan.

3. Bake 20 to 25 minutes or until lightly browned. Cool completely in pan on wire rack. Cut into 16 bars. Drizzle with melted chocolate. *Makes 16 bars*

Nutrients per Serving: *1 bar*
Calories: 91, **Calories from Fat:** 41%, **Total Fat:** 4g,
Saturated Fat: 1g, **Cholesterol:** <1mg, **Sodium:** 24mg,
Carbohydrate: 11g, **Fiber:** 1g, **Protein:** 3g

TIP   Flax seeds are an excellent source of omega-3 fatty acids, which may reduce the risk of heart disease. If you can't find flax seeds at the supermarket, look for them in a health food store. You can grind them in a coffee mill or blender.

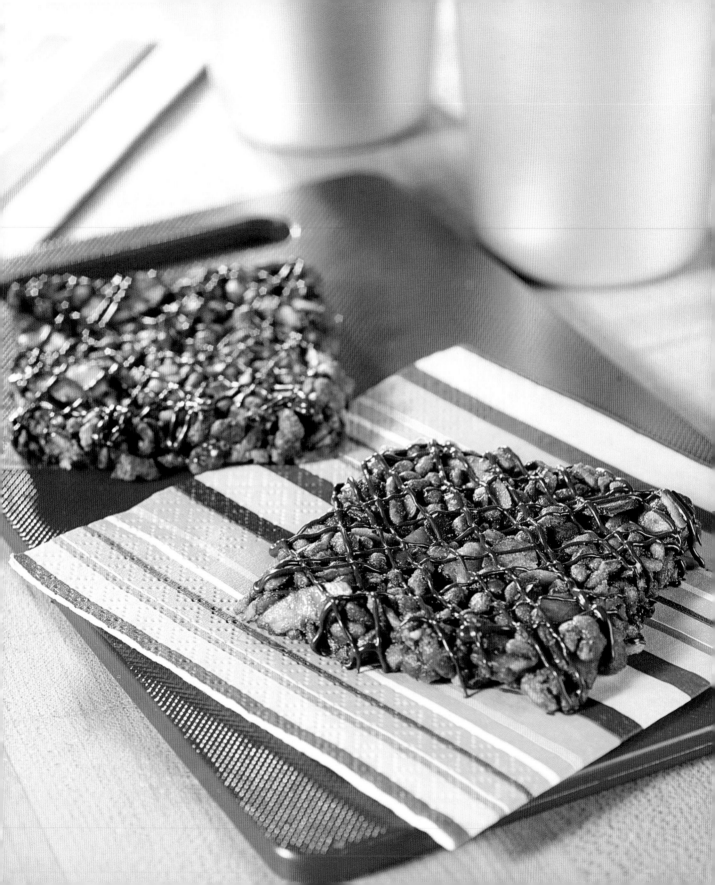

CHUNKY VEGGIE DIP

1 medium red bell pepper, chopped
1 large green bell pepper, chopped
½ medium onion, finely chopped
1 celery stalk, chopped
2 tablespoons water
⅛ teaspoon red pepper flakes
¼ cup fat-free (skim) milk
¾ teaspoon cornstarch
1 cup (4 ounces) shredded reduced-fat sharp Cheddar cheese
2 ounces reduced-fat cream cheese
1 jar (4 ounces) diced pimientos
¾ teaspoon salt
   Baked corn tortilla chips

Slow Cooker Directions

1. Spray slow cooker with nonstick cooking spray. Add bell peppers, onion, celery, water and red pepper flakes. Cover; cook on LOW 3 hours or until celery is tender.

2. Whisk milk and cornstarch in small bowl until smooth and well blended. Stir into slow cooker with Cheddar cheese and cream cheese until well blended and cheese is melted. Stir in pimientos and salt. Cover; cook on LOW 15 minutes or until thickened. Serve with tortilla chips, if desired.

Makes 12 servings

Nutrients per Serving: *¼ cup*
Calories: 47, **Calories from Fat:** 49%, **Total Fat:** 3g,
Saturated Fat: 2g, **Cholesterol:** 9mg, **Sodium:** 254mg,
Carbohydrate: 3g, **Fiber:** 1g, **Protein:** 3g

Variation: Use soft corn tortillas instead of chips. Cut each tortilla into 6 wedges and bake in single layer on baking sheet at 350°F for 10 minutes. Cool completely before serving. Chips will get crisp as they cool.

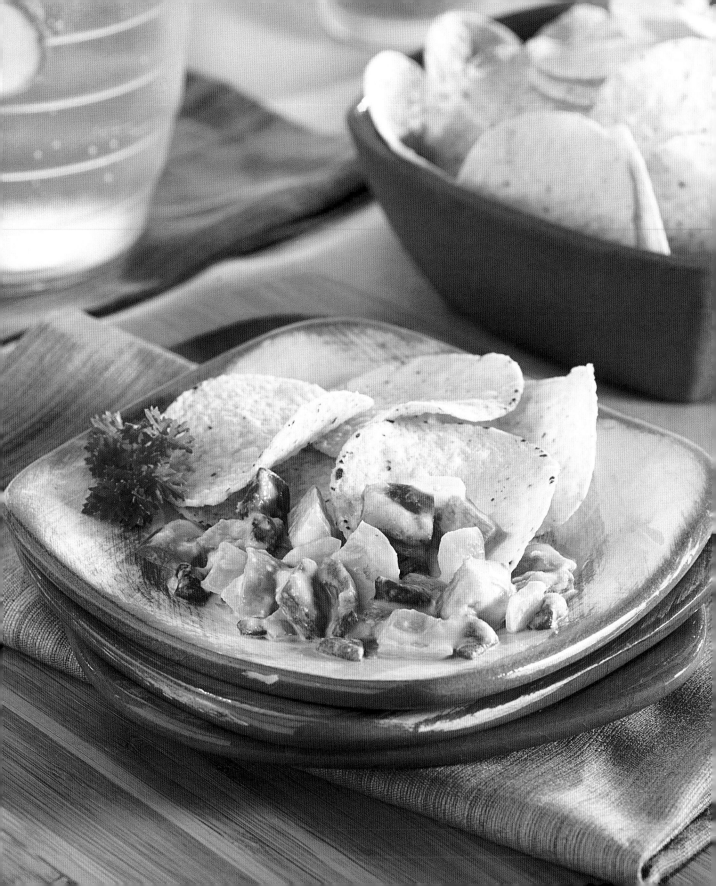

CRISP OATS TRAIL MIX

  1 cup old-fashioned oats
  ½ cup raw pumpkin seeds
  ½ cup dried sweetened cranberries
  ½ cup raisins
  2 tablespoons maple syrup
  1 teaspoon canola oil
  ½ teaspoon ground cinnamon
  ¼ teaspoon salt

1. Preheat oven to 325°F. Line baking sheet with heavy-duty foil.

2. Combine all ingredients in large bowl; mix well. Spread on prepared baking sheet.

3. Bake 20 minutes or until oats are lightly browned, stirring halfway through. Cool completely on baking sheet. Store in airtight container.

Makes 2½ cups (about 10 servings)

Nutrients per Serving: *¼ cup*
Calories: 123, **Calories from Fat:** 31%, **Total Fat:** 5g,
Saturated Fat: <1g, **Cholesterol:** 0mg, **Sodium:** 60mg,
Carbohydrate: 20g, **Fiber:** 2g, **Protein:** 3g

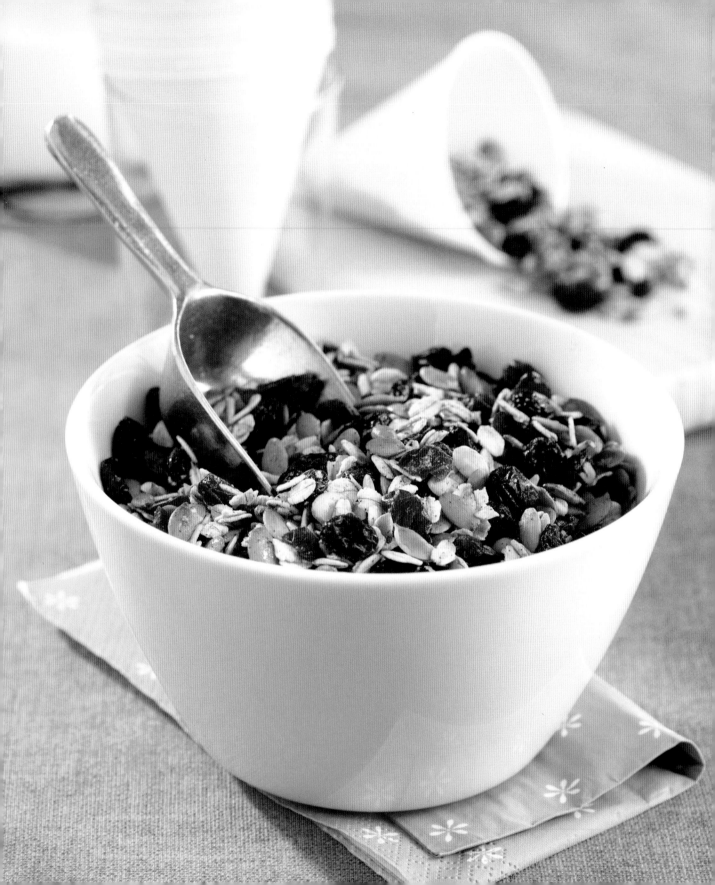

HERBED STUFFED TOMATOES

15 cherry tomatoes
½ cup low-fat (1%) cottage cheese
1 tablespoon thinly sliced green onion
1 teaspoon chopped fresh chervil *or* **¼ teaspoon dried chervil leaves**
½ teaspoon snipped fresh dill *or* **⅛ teaspoon dried dill weed**
⅛ teaspoon lemon pepper

1. Cut thin slice off bottom of each tomato. Scoop out pulp with small spoon; discard pulp. Invert tomatoes onto paper towels to drain.

2. Stir cottage cheese, green onion, chervil, dill and lemon pepper in small bowl until just combined. Spoon evenly into tomatoes. Serve immediately or cover and refrigerate up to 8 hours.
Makes 5 servings

Nutrients per Serving: *3 stuffed tomatoes*
Calories: 27, **Calories from Fat:** 12%, **Total Fat:** <1g,
Saturated Fat: <1g, **Cholesterol:** 1mg, **Sodium:** 96mg,
Carbohydrate: 3g, **Fiber:** <1g, **Protein:** 3g

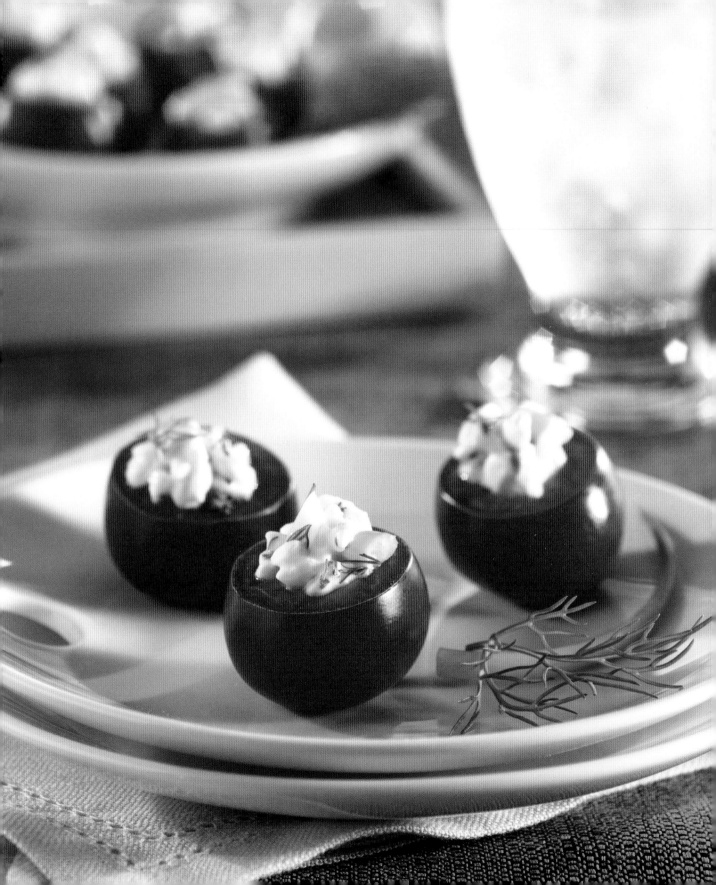

SAVORY PITA CHIPS

2 whole wheat or white pita bread rounds
   Olive oil cooking spray
3 tablespoons grated Parmesan cheese
1 teaspoon dried basil
¼ teaspoon garlic powder

1. Preheat oven to 350°F. Line baking sheet with foil.

2. Carefully cut each pita horizontally to split and form two rounds. Cut each round into six wedges.

3. Arrange wedges, rough sides down, in single layer on prepared baking sheet. Spray with cooking spray. Turn over; spray with cooking spray.

4. Combine cheese, basil and garlic powder in small bowl; sprinkle evenly over pita wedges.

5. Bake 12 to 14 minutes or until crisp and golden brown. Cool completely.

Makes 4 servings

Nutrients per Serving: *6 chips*
Calories: 108, **Calories from Fat:** 18%, **Total Fat:** 2g,
Saturated Fat: 1g, **Cholesterol:** 4mg, **Sodium:** 257mg,
Carbohydrate: 18g, **Fiber:** 2g, **Protein:** 5g

Cinnamon Crisps: Substitute butter-flavored cooking spray for the olive oil cooking spray and 1 tablespoon sugar mixed with ¼ teaspoon ground cinnamon for the Parmesan cheese, basil and garlic powder.

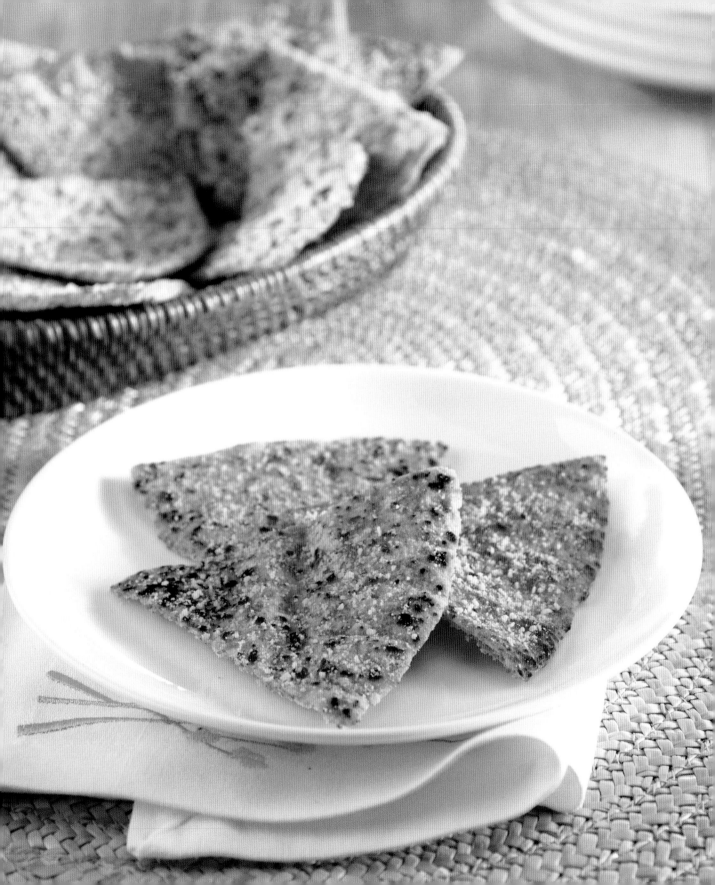

TRAIL MIX TRUFFLES

⅓ cup dried apples
¼ cup dried apricots
¼ cup apple butter
2 tablespoons golden raisins
1 tablespoon reduced-fat peanut butter
½ cup reduced-fat granola
¼ cup graham cracker crumbs, divided
¼ cup mini chocolate chips
1 tablespoon water

1. Combine apples, apricots, apple butter, raisins and peanut butter in food processor or blender; process until smooth. Stir in granola, 1 tablespoon graham cracker crumbs, chocolate chips and water until well combined. Shape into 16 balls.

2. Place remaining crumbs in shallow dish; roll balls in crumbs. Cover and refrigerate until ready to serve.

Makes 16 truffles

Nutrients per Serving: *2 truffles*
Calories: 121, **Calories from Fat:** 30%, **Total Fat:** 4g,
Saturated Fat: 1g, **Cholesterol:** 0mg, **Sodium:** 14mg,
Carbohydrate: 20g, **Fiber:** 2g, **Protein:** 3g

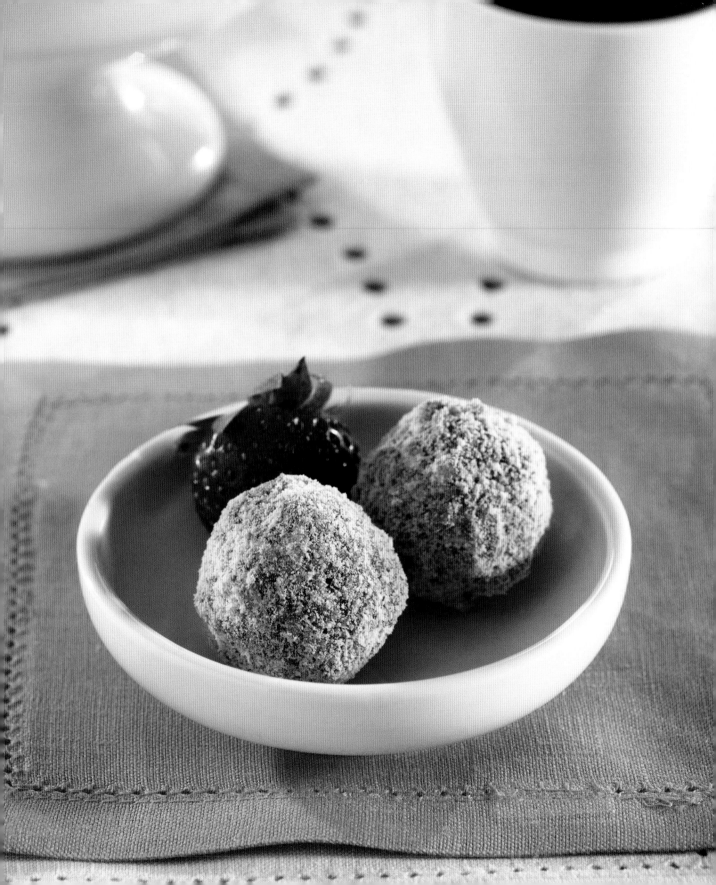

SPICY ROASTED CHICKPEAS

1 can (about 15 ounces) chickpeas, rinsed and drained
3 tablespoons olive oil
½ teaspoon salt
½ teaspoon black pepper
¾ to 1 tablespoon chili powder
⅛ to ¼ teaspoon ground red pepper
1 lime, cut into wedges

1. Preheat oven to 400°F.

2. Combine chickpeas, oil, salt and black pepper in large bowl. Spread in single layer on 15×10-inch jelly-roll pan.

3. Bake 15 minutes or until chickpeas begin to brown, shaking pan twice. Sprinkle with chili powder and red pepper. Bake 5 minutes or until dark golden-red. Serve with lime wedges.   *Makes 4 servings*

Nutrients per Serving: *½ cup*
Calories: 264, **Calories from Fat:** 40%, **Total Fat:** 12g,
Saturated Fat: 2g, **Cholesterol:** 0mg, **Sodium:** 730mg,
Carbohydrate: 33g, **Fiber:** 7g, **Protein:** 7g

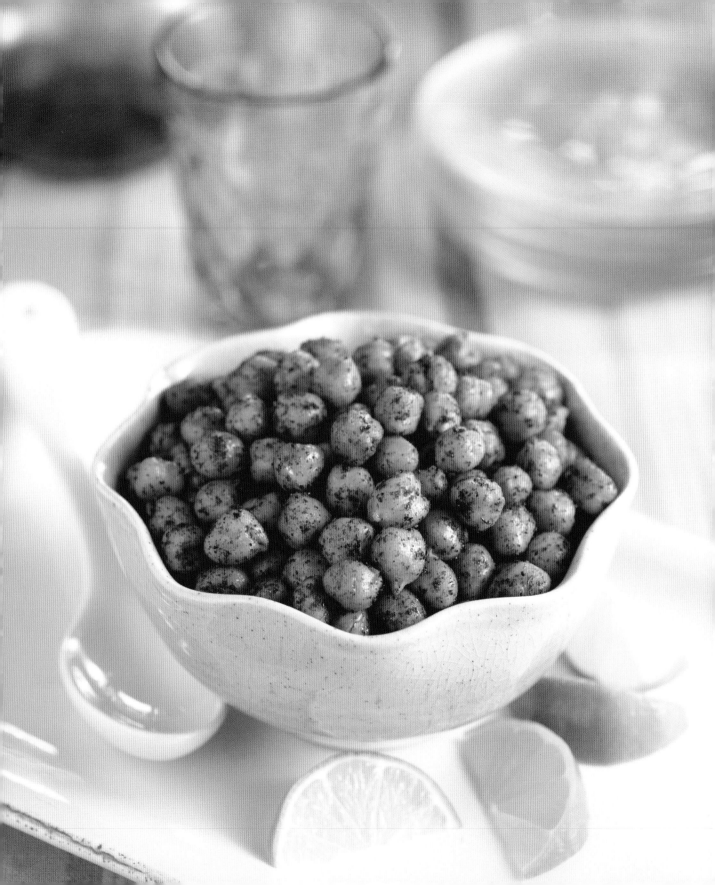

MEDITERRANEAN PITA PIZZAS

2 white or whole wheat pita bread rounds

1 teaspoon olive oil

1 cup canned cannellini beans, rinsed and drained

2 teaspoons lemon juice

2 cloves garlic, minced

½ cup thinly sliced radicchio or escarole lettuce (optional)

½ cup chopped tomato

½ cup finely chopped red onion

¼ cup (1 ounce) crumbled feta cheese

2 tablespoons sliced pitted black olives

1. Preheat oven to 450°F. Arrange pitas on baking sheet; brush tops with oil. Bake 6 minutes.

2. Meanwhile, place beans in small bowl; mash lightly with fork. Stir in lemon juice and garlic.

3. Spread bean mixture evenly on pita bread rounds to within ½ inch of edge. Top evenly with radicchio, if desired, tomato, onion, cheese and olives.

4. Bake 5 minutes or until heated through and crisp. To serve, cut each pizza into four wedges.

Makes 8 servings

Nutrients per Serving: *1 pizza wedge*
Calories: 98, **Calories from Fat:** 29%, **Total Fat:** 3g,
Saturated Fat: 1g, **Cholesterol:** 7mg, **Sodium:** 282mg,
Carbohydrate: 14g, **Fiber:** 2g, **Protein:** 4g

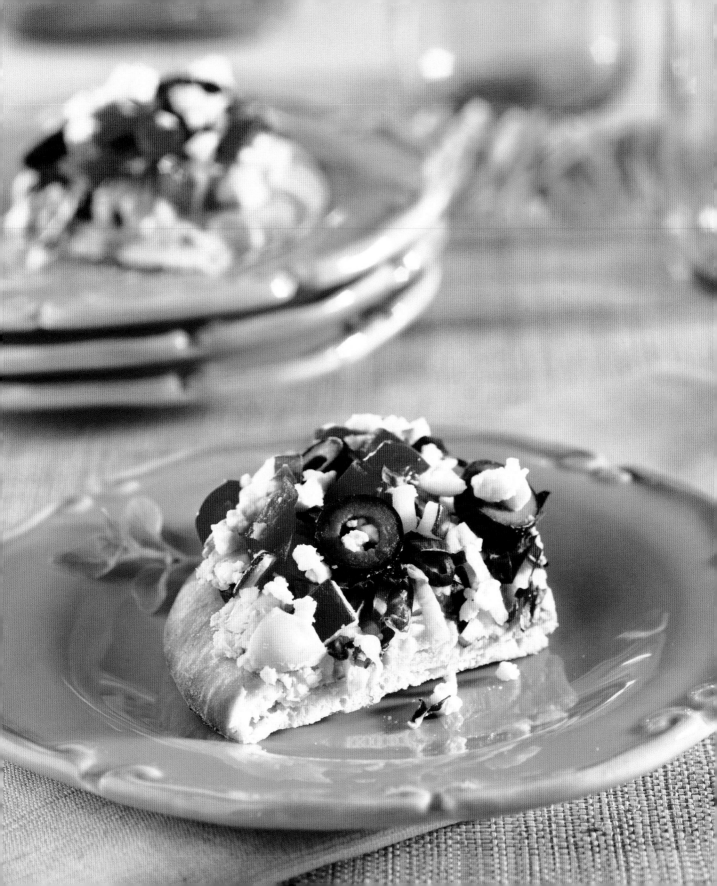

DILLY DEVILED EGGS

6 hard-cooked eggs, peeled and sliced in half lengthwise
1 tablespoon reduced-fat sour cream
1 tablespoon low-fat mayonnaise
1 tablespoon low-fat (1%) cottage cheese
1 tablespoon minced fresh dill *or* 1 teaspoon dried dill weed
1 tablespoon minced dill pickle
1 teaspoon Dijon mustard
⅛ teaspoon salt
⅛ teaspoon ground white pepper
  Paprika (optional)
  Dill sprigs (optional)

1. Remove yolks from egg halves. Mash yolks with sour cream, mayonnaise, cottage cheese, dill, pickle, mustard, salt and white pepper in small bowl.

2. Using teaspoon or piping bag fitted with large plain tip, fill egg halves with mixture. Sprinkle with paprika, if desired. Garnish with dill sprigs.   *Makes 6 servings*

Nutrients per Serving: *2 egg halves*
Calories: 93, **Calories from Fat:** 64%, **Total Fat:** 6g,
Saturated Fat: 2g, **Cholesterol:** 214mg, **Sodium:** 177mg,
Carbohydrate: 1g, **Fiber:** <1g, **Protein:** 7g

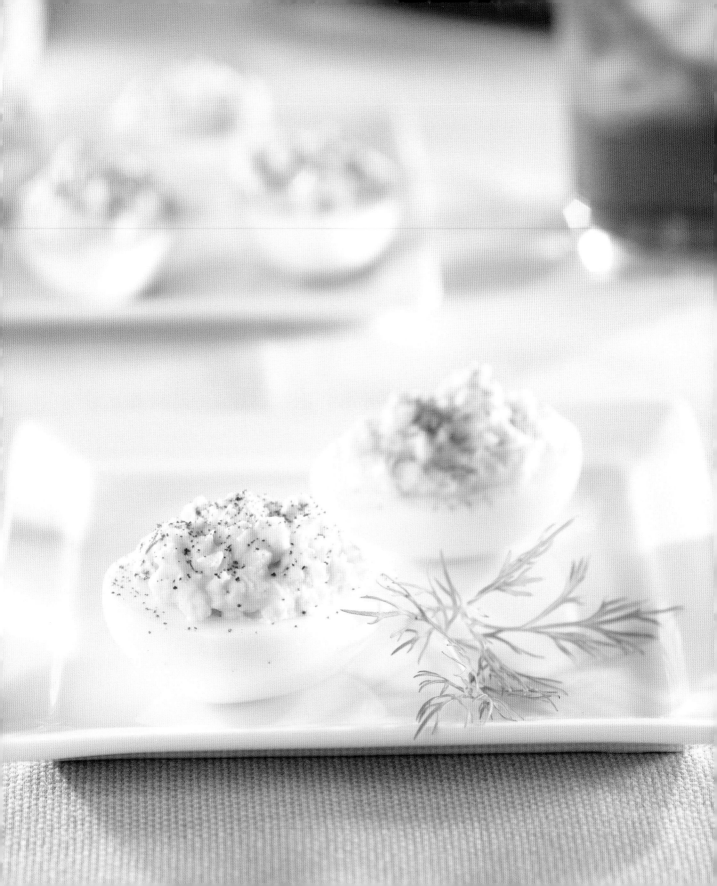

COCONUT ALMOND BISCOTTI

2½ cups all-purpose flour

1⅓ cups unsweetened shredded coconut

¾ cup sliced almonds

⅔ cup sugar

2 teaspoons baking powder

½ teaspoon salt

1 egg

1 egg white

½ cup (1 stick) butter, melted

1 teaspoon vanilla

1. Preheat to 350°F. Line baking sheet with parchment paper.

2. Combine flour, coconut, almonds, sugar, baking powder and salt in large bowl; mix well. Beat egg, egg white, butter and vanilla in medium bowl. Add to flour mixture; mix with electric mixer at low speed until blended.

3. Divide dough evenly into two pieces. Shape each piece into 8×2¾-inch loaf with lightly floured hands. Place loaves 3 inches apart on prepared baking sheet.

4. Bake 26 to 28 minutes or until golden and set. Cool on baking sheet on wire rack 10 minutes.

5. Using serrated knife, slice each loaf diagonally into ½-inch-thick slices. Place slices, cut sides down, on baking sheet. Bake 20 minutes or until firm and golden. Cool completely on wire rack.

Makes about 2 dozen biscotti

Nutrients per Serving: *1 biscotti*
Calories: 126, **Calories from Fat:** 45%, **Total Fat:** 6g,
Saturated Fat: 3g, **Cholesterol:** 14mg, **Sodium:** 68mg,
Carbohydrate: 15g, **Fiber:** 1g, **Protein:** 3g

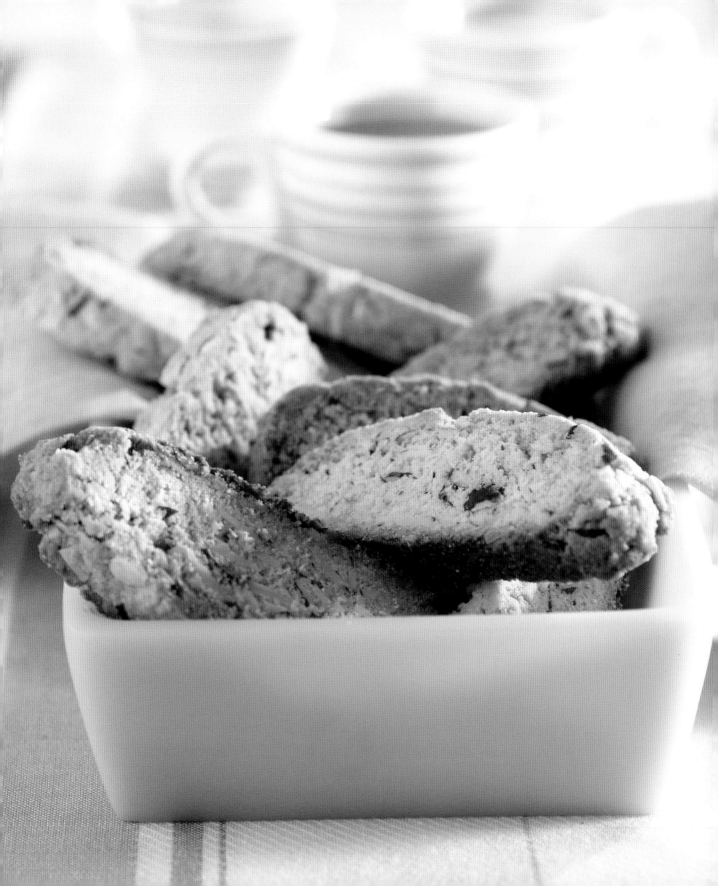

METRIC CONVERSION CHART

VOLUME MEASUREMENTS (dry)

$1/8$ teaspoon = 0.5 mL
$1/4$ teaspoon = 1 mL
$1/2$ teaspoon = 2 mL
$3/4$ teaspoon = 4 mL
1 teaspoon = 5 mL
1 tablespoon = 15 mL
2 tablespoons = 30 mL
$1/4$ cup = 60 mL
$1/3$ cup = 75 mL
$1/2$ cup = 125 mL
$2/3$ cup = 150 mL
$3/4$ cup = 175 mL
1 cup = 250 mL
2 cups = 1 pint = 500 mL
3 cups = 750 mL
4 cups = 1 quart = 1 L

VOLUME MEASUREMENTS (fluid)

1 fluid ounce (2 tablespoons) = 30 mL
4 fluid ounces ($1/2$ cup) = 125 mL
8 fluid ounces (1 cup) = 250 mL
12 fluid ounces ($1 1/2$ cups) = 375 mL
16 fluid ounces (2 cups) = 500 mL

WEIGHTS (mass)

$1/2$ ounce = 15 g
1 ounce = 30 g
3 ounces = 90 g
4 ounces = 120 g
8 ounces = 225 g
10 ounces = 285 g
12 ounces = 360 g
16 ounces = 1 pound = 450 g

DIMENSIONS

$1/16$ inch = 2 mm
$1/8$ inch = 3 mm
$1/4$ inch = 6 mm
$1/2$ inch = 1.5 cm
$3/4$ inch = 2 cm
1 inch = 2.5 cm

OVEN TEMPERATURES

250°F = 120°C
275°F = 140°C
300°F = 150°C
325°F = 160°C
350°F = 180°C
375°F = 190°C
400°F = 200°C
425°F = 220°C
450°F = 230°C

BAKING PAN SIZES

Utensil	Size in Inches/Quarts	Metric Volume	Size in Centimeters
Baking or Cake Pan (square or rectangular)	$8 \times 8 \times 2$	2 L	$20 \times 20 \times 5$
	$9 \times 9 \times 2$	2.5 L	$23 \times 23 \times 5$
	$12 \times 8 \times 2$	3 L	$30 \times 20 \times 5$
	$13 \times 9 \times 2$	3.5 L	$33 \times 23 \times 5$
Loaf Pan	$8 \times 4 \times 3$	1.5 L	$20 \times 10 \times 7$
	$9 \times 5 \times 3$	2 L	$23 \times 13 \times 7$
Round Layer Cake Pan	$8 \times 1 1/2$	1.2 L	20×4
	$9 \times 1 1/2$	1.5 L	23×4
Pie Plate	$8 \times 1 1/4$	750 mL	20×3
	$9 \times 1 1/4$	1 L	23×3
Baking Dish or Casserole	1 quart	1 L	—
	$1 1/2$ quart	1.5 L	—
	2 quart	2 L	—